AUTHORITATIVE AND
GUT REACTIONS TELLS YOU:

—the key differences between stress-symptoms and signs of organic disease

—the physical changes in your body when you're having a gut reaction

—personality characteristics of gut reactors

—how to select a doctor—and why you must take ultimate responsibility for your own health

—the medical tests that may be necessary to rule out organic disease—exactly what will happen and the purpose of each test

—tips for coping with everyday stress—and how to handle the major life changes that are likely to affect your stomach

David M. Taylor, M.D., is director of the Gastro-intestinal Diagnostic Unit at Georgia Baptist Hospital and Northside Hospital in Atlanta. **Maxine A. Rock** has published over 100 lay medical and scientific articles and has received nine academic and professional awards for her science writing.

GUT REACTIONS
HOW TO HANDLE
STRESS
AND YOUR
STOMACH

David M. Taylor, M.D. / Maxine A. Rock

BERKLEY BOOKS, NEW YORK

THIS BOOK IS DEDICATED
TO OUR FAMILIES AND FRIENDS,
WHO HAD THE GUTS
TO SEE US THROUGH.

This Berkley book contains the complete
text of the original hardcover edition.
It has been completely reset in a typeface
designed for easy reading, and was printed
from new film

GUT REACTIONS

A Berkley Book / published by arrangement with
the Saunders Press

PRINTING HISTORY
Saunders Press edition published 1980
Berkley edition / January 1983
Second printing / July 1983

ISBN: 0-425-05635-X

A BERKLEY BOOK ® TM 757,375
Berkley Books are published by The Berkley Publishing Group,
200 Madison Avenue, New York, New York 10016.
The name "BERKLEY" and the stylized "B" with design
are trademarks belonging to Berkley Publishing Corporation.
PRINTED IN THE UNITED STATES OF AMERICA

Acknowledgments

We acknowledge with thanks and affection the special help, encouragement, and wisdom given by David Rock; Arlene Taylor gets applause, too, for her composure; as does Jean Hochman, who helped with home-cooked meals; and our children—Howard, Debbie, and Robyn Taylor, and Lauren and Michael Rock—who provided understanding, patience, and comic relief.

We thank Peggy Hood who did a marvelous job typing the final draft of the manuscript, offering assistance when the going got rough, and we also offer appreciation to Nancy Adams and Faye Johnson for their typing and clerical work.

Doctors David Hein and Bob Goldstein should get awards because they're still smiling at their partner, David Taylor. We are also grateful to Dr. Eddy Palmer for his thoughtful reading of our manuscript. And, we both thank all the patients and other doctors who willingly talked to Maxine and contributed their stories and experiences for use in this book.

Contents

Preface

This book was born over a plate of spicy spaghetti sauce. It started about noon on a sunny Monday in June, 1978, when I was having lunch with my doctor and friend, David Taylor. I still remember the sharp, satisfying taste of the sauce; the soft scuffing of nurses' crepe-soled shoes on the floor of the Georgia Baptist Hospital cafeteria; the curious mixture of food smells, and the starchy scent of doctors' white examining coats.

David and I, hunched over our food, were talking about my remarkable "recovery" from functional gastrointestinal disease. For eight years—ever since I came to a new career and a new life in Atlanta in 1969—he and I had been trying to deal with my frequent and terrifying bouts of stomach pain, nausea, and diarrhea. The symptoms often pulled me, a self-employed journalist, away from lunch with clients or stabbed at me while I was in my car zooming toward a story. The pain confused and frightened me, and it was costing a fortune in medical bills. It worried my husband and spoiled good times with my two young children.

When I first came to David with the symptoms and he pronounced me physically healthy, I remember looking at him with tears in my eyes and saying, "That may be so . . . but until I get rid of these gut problems. I'm crippled."

I *did* get rid of them, but it wasn't easy. David and I hunted together for answers, and often we found only frustration. I boiled with questions, sometimes asking the same ones over and over. If I wasn't *sick*, why was I in pain? What was happening to my body when the symptoms hit? If this wasn't just "all in my head," why couldn't David cure me? Why take test after test if David was really sure I was okay? And, how could I be *okay* if I felt miserable so often?

David probed, examined, checked his notes, took more tests, and again answered my questions. Much of the time he *had* no answers. I was expecting a diagnosis, a prescription, and a cure. But often all I saw was David's silent smile and a shrug of his shoulders.

It took me a while to learn that David was being honest. Functional gastrointestinal disease doesn't lend itself to easy answers. We experimented hundreds of times with different medicines, diets, and exercises. I endured X-rays, sonar bounces, lighted tubes stuck down my throat, and many other uncomfortable, undignified, and expensive diagnostic tests. Several times I landed in the hospital with uncontrollable spasms. David would come to my room, sit at the side of my bed, and rub his black goatee like a general who is planning war.

"Now we'll try this . . ." he'd say. And we always tried. We were both much too determined to give up.

Over the years that determination paid off. Gradually I discovered that the spasms and other gut symptoms were my deeply disguised method of reacting to stress. The stress didn't have to come in the form of unpleasant events. Sometimes an unexpected invitation to dinner or a minor change in my schedule could erupt into a giant bellyache. The pain might move elusively from one spot to another. It might be fleeting, or last for hours. Seemingly, it did not connect itself to any one event, but if I kept tabs on how I *felt* about that event, I could usually associate bottled-up anger, confusion, or even joy with an eventual gut reaction. So I started using the phrase "gut reaction" when I wanted to tell David that I suspected I was having pain because I was upset or excited about something.

The reaction wasn't always immediate, either. Sometimes I'd do fine during a crisis, then crumple with pain a few weeks or even a few months later. Within the same month my father died, my daughter was born, and I hurt my back in an accident, and friends were amazed at how well I "stood up." I kept working and smiling; I wanted to be strong, so I could comfort and care for my family. (I should have sobbed, and let out my confusion and grief!) My self-control lasted almost a year, but the charade finally cost me such intense gut pain that David was forced to make a rush visit to my house. I was pale and skinny and frightened; he was flushed, fighting to stay calm. His lean face was twisted with sympathy and frustration. He threw his stethoscope on the bed and bellowed, "Max, you are *not* sick. We will beat this thing yet!"

This book is about how we "beat" functional gastrointestinal disease. David and I both thought of writing the book almost at the same moment: the day we had lunch to celebrate our victory. I scooped up my spaghetti sauce, and said, "It's so great to eat this stuff, and not worry about it. It's so great to be free!" David held his fork in midair and looked at me. We both laughed. "This is an anniversary," he said, waving the fork with excitement. "It's been one whole year since you've had any problems with your guts."

"If they ever do come again we can handle them," I rejoined, clinking my fork with David's, and spattering tiny red globs of sauce on his tie. "I hope all your patients can say that some day."

We both laughed again, because we said simultaneously, "Let's write a book."

Here's how we went about it: At the start of each new chapter, David and I discussed what needed to be said about our specific subject, such as diet and drugs, life-style, and so on. Then we compared our research, and David dictated a rough draft of the chapter, in medical jargon. I rewrote what he said to help lay people understand it, added case histories from David's files and from my own experience, and pumped other doctors for more opinions and information. David's personality is present throughout the book because the "I" in the book is his voice, the voice of medical authority. It is enough for me to tell you here that my experience is deeply entwined with every word.

By the time you have finished reading it, I hope you'll feel that this book is true to your own experience. Each chapter is intended to send you the message that no patient can be a passive partner in his own "cure." If you want to control your gut reactions, as I did, you will have to take the lead: arm yourself with information about your disease; insist on a doctor who shares your belief in the possibility for a symptom-free life and who isn't afraid to keep trying; and be prepared to cooperate fully and enthusiastically with that doctor over a long period of time. You will be the one doing most of the work, but you'll also reap most of the rewards (including spaghetti sauce).

Responsibility for freedom from any disease is, I believe, mostly up to you.

Maxine A. Rock
Atlanta, Georgia
April, 1980

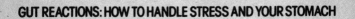
GUT REACTIONS: HOW TO HANDLE STRESS AND YOUR STOMACH

Introduction

People come to doctors most often when they have health problems they can't understand or handle alone. Perhaps one of the most frustrating of these problems—for both patient and physician—is symptomatic gut distress, which commonly shows up as constantly churning intestines, stomach pain, heartburn, nausea, weakness, bloating, and gas. These are the pains of the so-called "irritable gut syndrome."

Doctors struggle to recognize this very common syndrome because it is displayed in so many different ways by so many different kinds of patients, most of whom are otherwise healthy. Often when a doctor does make the proper diagnosis, he can't or won't take the time to explore the disorder with his baffled patient, study the problem, explain the difference between serious organic disease and non-serious, but painful functional disorders, and then treat each new and stubborn symptom until it disappears or subsides enough to let the patient go on with his life.

Many patients, too, are puzzled by the painful and annoying symptoms that their doctors might tell them are "all in your head." That phrase, which is repeated every day by overworked doctors to trembling and then humiliated patients in thousands of examining rooms all over the country, suggests that the irritable gut syndrome is an imaginary problem, or that the patient is faking his symptoms. That's not true. Real bodily changes are occurring when you feel a gut symptom, and the disorder is as real and as crippling as a broken bone. What the doctor probably means to say is that the *cause* of your irritable gut symptoms is emotional even though the *result* is physical. Emotional upheaval is affecting your digestive tract, and the pain, vomiting, and other symptoms can be perceived as distress signals coming from the area you generally call your stomach.

You can't ignore those signals; they hurt too much. But you *can* recognize and fight them, and win. That's what this book is all about.

Doctors say mysterious gut dysfunctions plague millions of Americans. Just think of all the times you've missed work or social functions because your stomach was "upset"; how often you have heard youngsters beg to stay home from school because "my tummy hurts"; or how common it is to express sympathy to a friend who admits he can't deliver an important speech or perform on the job because "my guts are churning." According to A. A. Chaplan, a physician and psychiatrist at New York's French–Polyclinic Medical

School, the gastrointestinal tract has become the "target organ" for physical distress stemming from emotional upheaval. The distress often reaches gigantic proportions; since about 1940, claims Dr. Chaplan, bellyaches have been filling more United States hospital beds than any other "disease." In April, 1969, an article appeared in the medical journal *Viewpoints on Digestive Diseases* noting that digestive disorders are this nation's "principal cause of physical suffering, loss of time from work, and economic disability."

Still doctors and patients don't know much about these and other psychosomatic disabilities, though they have been recognized at least since Hippocrates. That ancient father of medicine noted the link between emotional and physical suffering in saying, "The common knowledge [is] that man gets sick when life circumstances are adverse, and is healthy when they are propitious." As early as 3200 B.C. the Greeks and Egyptians found that emotional disturbances were often followed by a physical breakdown of one sort or another, while the Old-World Hebrews insisted that sickness was God's punishment for breaking religious laws. Both Plato and Aristotle wrote that feelings of anger or joy had an effect on the body. Thousands of years later the pioneer of psychotherapy, Sigmund Freud, discovered that he could cure patients of paralysis and other physical diseases by allowing them to vent and understand their repressed emotions.

Specific research linking gut pain to emotional turmoil has been going on since 1822. On June 6th of that year, a freak accident happened at a remote trading post on Mackinac Island, Michigan. Alexis

St. Martin, a nineteen-year-old boy, was chatting with some friends at the trading post when someone tripped over a shotgun. The shotgun discharged and blew a huge hole in St. Martin's stomach. The youth fell down screaming, his shirt on fire, and while he lay suffering, bystanders saw that the food St. Martin had for breakfast that morning was pouring out of the hole. Fortunately, William Beaumont, an army doctor, was one of those bystanders. He treated St. Martin and saved his life.

But the stomach wound never healed. It was an "open window" on St. Martin's churning guts. Dr. Beaumont persuaded the grateful patient to let him peer through that window—in the name of science—for a number of years.

By looking directly into St. Martin's stomach as it worked, Dr. Beaumont learned that food is broken down by gastric juices, that stomachs "growl" when they are empty because air swooshes around inside them, and that the stomach behaved in strange ways when St. Martin was upset. Dr. Beaumont thus made the first recorded, scientific, direct connection between the gastrointestinal tract and emotional distress.

Another doctor, together with another unfortunate boy, inadvertently continued the research in 1895. The boy, who was nine years old, was simply known as "Tom." One hot day in 1895, Tom tried to sneak a mouthful of what he thought was cool beer, when his dad's back was turned. But what he really gulped was searing hot clam chowder, which his father had carried home in a beer pail. The chowder burned Tom's esophagus. The only way he could live was for doctors to make a hole directly into his stomach by performing a surgical procedure known as a gastrostomy, so that food could be poured into his stomach through a funnel.

Tom lived with his "hole" for many years. Since it was a great handicap it was difficult for Tom to find work. So, when a curious young doctor and medical researcher named Stuart Wolf offered Tom a job as a "research subject," Tom jumped at the chance. Tom earned his money by performing some janitorial chores around the laboratory, and by letting Dr. Wolf occasionally look into his stomach.

When Dr. Wolf looked, he found that Tom's stomach, like ours, changed with Tom's moods. "[The stomach] membrane became scarlet and turgid during excitement or anger, brought on most often by a slight, real or imagined, to Tom's competence or conscientiousness," Dr. Wolfe later wrote. "When Tom was frightened or depressed, usually because of fear of losing his job, the [stomach] membrane turned pale, dry, thin, and sticky. The changes in the mucosa were often correlated with changes in the color of his face. Thus, at times, when he was red in the face and 'hot under the collar,' his stomach was likely to be red and turgid. On the other hand, when Tom was pale and listless, his stomach was correspondingly pallid."

Tom made medical history: his most important contribution to science, according to Dr. Wolf, was to show doctors the significant relationship "between emotions and visceral function." Dr. Wolf was so impressed with that relationship that he wrote a book about it called *The Stomach*. The book, published by Oxford University Press, tells what Dr. Wolf learned from Tom, and sums up Dr. Wolf's feeling that the stomach is "the seat of the soul and still a recognized source of ecstasy and grief."

From the studies done on Alexis St. Martin and Tom, doctors know that emotional problems cause real bodily changes, such as intestinal spasm and secretion, variations in blood chemistry levels, and hormonal secretions. Doctors are also reminded through more recent reports and studies that patients can't easily control these symptoms. In 1976, for example, a study at the Mayo Clinic showed that chronic nausea could be a "face-saving maneuver," but patients who used nausea as a social weapon didn't really know what they were doing or how they were doing it. It is also generally recognized, but not scientifically proven, that patients with functional gastrointestinal symptoms cannot control those symptoms unless specifically trained to do so, and that the symptoms can change if the patient's emotional environment changes. The doctor–patient relationship can also affect the symptoms, for better or worse, but it is often impossible to find out *how* this happens.

So for the most part, the "irritable colon," "spastic bowel," or the "overactive gastrointestinal tract" remains a mystery. It's such a frustrating medical problem that some doctors may try to ignore it and send the patient away, or treat the symptoms with never-ending doses of tranquilizers. Other doctors simply tell a patient, "It's all in your head." We've already said it's not. The churning, pain, bloating, and other symptoms are real, and they are enough to cripple some people. Sometimes the crippling effect of the symptoms makes people ashamed of themselves for having these symptoms, and thus "displaying" their emotional problems to the world. It also makes them think they are not "worthy" of medical care. Dr. George Silver, Professor of Public Health at Yale University's School of Medicine, said in his 1976 book, *A Spy In The House of Medicine,* that many people won't level with their doctors because they fear "the doctor is contemptuous of their symptoms, that they are not really sick, that he thinks that it is all in their heads." Alexander Solzhenitsyn echoes this fear in his novel *Cancer Ward*, when one his characters, an old family doctor, asks, "How many adult human beings are there, now, at this minute, rushing about in mute panic wishing they could find a doctor, the kind of person to whom they could pour out the fears they have deeply concealed or even found shameful?"

People who are sick are frequently afraid. When you are a gut reactor, you must add to that fear an additional worry: that you are "crazy," as well, because your sickness appears to have no physical base. And, of course, you also suspect that your doctor may think you are faking. But you should know that in October, 1969, the medical journal *Lancet* described a year-long study of patients with the irritable bowel syndrome, which provided information showing that gut symptoms were the result of definite body changes, and that patients didn't—and couldn't—"fake" or "imagine" those symptoms. The study didn't show patients how to cure the symptoms, but the people involved in the study were so hungry for information concerning their disorder that even though the study couldn't tell them how to get better, a doctor said that "Many [patients with gut symptoms] expressed their gratitude that someone had at last made an attempt to understand them and did not regard their symptoms as imaginary."

Dr. Eddy Palmer, one of this nation's most respected gastric specialists, lamented in his classic doctor's manual, *Functional Gastrointestinal Disease*, that "gastritis studies are scarce and most are concerned with pathology and immunology . . . [We need] support for the concepts that anatomic changes of the gastric mucosa may be caused by emotional stress."

Not only do physical changes occur as a result of emotional problems, but those changes can manifest themselves in a variety of ways. Dr. S. Eugene Sims, a general surgeon and Southeast Medical Director of the Long Lines Division of American Telephone and Telegraph, says workers under stress show up in his office with headaches, muscle strain, blurred vision, colds, and backaches. But, he adds, "bellyaches" are the most common stress-linked disorders, and they can often keep an employee off the job for days. Atlanta gynecologist Dr. Michael Wolfson says that stress-induced pain can show up as vaginal ache, and that stress can definitely interfere with sexual drive and performance. In addition, he said, since cramping in the lower abdomen often is confused with menstrual pain, "It's amazing how many women come to a gynecologist and have functional abdominal complaints."

Even if doctors respect the "realness" of a patient's gut pain, they often don't know how to help. Dr. Palmer says managing gut symptoms "is one of the toughest jobs in medicine."

We hope this book will make the job easier, both for doctors and patients. The only way to beat gut reactions and keep a tight lid on the way stress affects your stomach is to understand the problem and the process. Then, working together, doctor and patient can find the way to a fuller, more pain-free life.

1

The Gut Reactor

There is no easy way to characterize gut reactors, because they pop up in every age group. People of both sexes and widely varying life-styles get emotional bellyaches. Some of them complain loudly about their painful guts; others suffer in relative silence. There's only one generalization doctors *can* make: chronic gut reactions signal stress.

The stress is well-hidden in most gut reactors. These people usually aren't hysterical, or "crazy-acting." Far from it! Patients with functional gut pain are most often well-organized, compulsive, bright, educated individuals who like to get things done—and done right. Trouble is, when things *don't* go right they become overly anxious and the anxiety is somaticized—"soma" means body—into a gut reaction. The anxiety turns into a bodily function.

All of us have physical reactions to anxiety from time to time; patients tell me, for example, that when they were suddenly startled "It felt like my stomach leapt up." That's normal, but a constantly leaping stomach means chronic depression, chronic anxiety, or both. This depression and anxiety may be subconscious, but it nevertheless is rocking your personal lifeboat. When the boat rocks, the guts heave. In some people, the heaving starts almost at birth.

Perhaps the best way to describe the kinds of people, young and old, who suffer this way is from the doctor's point of view. I'll start with Charlie. He was only nine months old when I saw him, but I knew that unless something changed fast, he was doomed to a lifetime of gut reactions.

Charlie was chubby, dark-haired, and full of life. He mouthed my stethoscope, yanked my beard, and slid the pen out of my shirt pocket and had me laughing at the way he rolled it across the examining table. But when he tried to crawl after the pen, Charlie's mother yelped and grabbed him. Did she think I'd let him tumble off and crack his skull? Clearly, she was jumpy, overprotective, and watched Charlie like a hawk.

"I've had him to doctors since he was four months old," she said. "He cries all the time. He spits up. His stomach is bloated. He has . . . uh . . . irregular bowel movements," she added, almost in a whisper. Then she sighed. She was young and well-dressed. Her heart-shaped face was pretty, except for the deep frown lines on her forehead and around her mouth.

"Charlie is just difficult to manage," she said at last. Then she sighed again.

Charlie seemed healthy enough to me. His height (24 inches) and weight (eighteen pounds) were normal. His fetal development and birth had been normal, and he was fed the usual infant diet of formula and strained food, then went on table food at seven months of age. When I poked his belly I found no bloated or misshapen organs, and all of Charlie's vital signs—heart, blood pressure, temperature, knee-jerk reactions—were good.

"He seems perfectly fine," I said. "Everything checks out." I tried to sound cheerful and reassuring. But Charlie's mother peered at me, and frowned. I tickled the baby's tummy and he laughed. "You're in for it, kiddo," I thought. "She's not going to be satisfied with that."

So in the next few days Charlie was whisked into the hospital laboratory for tests to see if he was absorbing his food normally; to see if he had any major organ disease; and to rule out any milk intolerance or allergies. His mother stoically obeyed all my orders. She called a few times to tell me Charlie was yowling a lot, but she never made a pest of herself. She was bright, concerned, and conscientious. I told her I'd yowl too, if I was Charlie and people in white caps were poking needles into me. She tried to chuckle.

After studying the lab results, I was left with a picture of a normal child whose mother had vague, colic-type complaints about him.

Charlie was having gut reactions to his nervous, fidgety mother. And unless she changed, Charlie was in for a lifetime of pain.

Two British doctors, John Apley and Barbara Hale, recently kept records on thirty children under the age of six who manifested what the doctors called "recurrent cryptic abdominal pain."

When the kids hit the age of twenty-four, it was found that two-thirds of them had been in and out of doctors' offices all their lives and still had that same gut pain. It didn't make any difference if the pain was treated or not; it came back anyway. Most of these patients came from "painful families," where one or both parents also complained of things like "irritable colon," "gas and bloating," or "lots of constipation." In a family atmosphere like this, said the doctors, the children hear gut complaints all the time and start some gut reactions of their own.

"Little bellyachers grow up to be big bellyachers," said the doctors.

Perhaps Charlie was already on his way.

So on the next visit Charlie's mother came alone. She told me she was a bacteriologist, but had stopped work to raise Charlie. Her husband was an attorney; he was just beginning practice and they were trying to establish themselves in a new community. Yes, she admitted, she was "uptight." Yes, she herself was a "colicky baby." Yes, her own doctor was treating her for "irritable colon."

"Look," I said, "this is a common problem. It's not Charlie's problem yet. It's yours. Charlie has what we'll call colic, for lack of a better term. His guts are churning because he's picking up on your nervousness. Kids need security, and who can feel secure around a nervous mother?"

Charlie's mother said softly, "I understand. What can I do?"

We started talking about how she might go back to work right now, and not hover over Charlie so much. I also wanted her to forget about those "irregular bowel movements" and let the kid dirty his diapers in his own good time. The central theme of the conversation was that if she loosened up and realized Charlie was a healthy baby, he'd probably stay that way.

When she left, Charlie's mother grabbed my hand and said she'd try to relax. I hope she did. I never saw Charlie again.

Children don't often come to a gastric specialist's office; pediatricians can usually handle their minor gut complaints. So I was surprised to see eight-year-old Sally, a first-grade student, a few days later. Sally said she'd been having "sore tummies" for two years. They started when she turned six and still persisted. The pain usually came on Monday or after a school holiday. Sally's biggest problem, she said shyly, was "going to the bathroom." She was constipation-prone, often went five or six days without a bowel movement, and once had a fecal impaction so severe it took oil enemas and manual manipulation to get relief. Her parents pumped drugstore laxatives into her. That often caused more tummy pain, Sally said, but it didn't help her much with the bowel movements.

I saw Sally alone in the examining room, although her mother (a school teacher) and her father (a business executive) hovered near the door. Sally didn't like my pressing and probing, but she was patient. She winced and her gray eyes filled with tears when I gave her a rectal exam. That's not much fun for doctors, either, but I had to do it. There was fecal material in there all right.

I ordered a series of tests for Sally: a proctoscopy, which is a procedure involving the insertion of a lighted tube into a patient's rectum to make sure there are no tumors or irritations in the tissues there; X-rays; blood studies to examine her metabolism, and a barium enema, to determine the shape and structure of the colon. All the test results showed Sally was fine.

But Sally wasn't fine. She was a testy, defensive little girl who once noticed with disdain that I had a stain on my tie. I told her it was spaghetti sauce from lunch and tried to make her laugh about it. But Sally wasn't amused. She tucked a strand of light brown hair into her tightly-coiled braids and said bluntly, "It's very important to be clean."

Sally had a passion for cleanliness. She insisted her mother clean the dining room daily, because Sally wailed "the food might get dirty!" She kept her own room perfect, never spilled anything at the table, and even wanted her jeans to be spotless.

Sally's parents encouraged what they called her "responsible attitude." Her father said, "We like to have things proper, too." Then he went on to tell me that Sally was a whiz at school and an "angel" at home. Her only problem was these terrible stomachaches.

Sally seemed to trust me a bit more the next time I saw her. She confided that things were "really terrible" at school because, she said, "I just hate to go to the bathroom any place except at home. The toilet seats are so dirty."

Later, I told Sally's folks that their preoccupation with neatness had transferred to Sally, and apparently was turning her into a kid who had to have everything under perfect control. Sally's father grimaced and said "I had a hunch it was something like that all along."

I told them to stop giving laxatives to Sally and feed her bran cereal instead; it's the best bulk agent. The trouble with nonnatural bowel stimulants is that they make the intestines do cartwheels, and this causes pain. Eventually the gut wall can't push the fecal matter along on its own power. The muscles get lazy because they're "addicted" to laxatives.

"What if bran doesn't help, and Sally still can't have a bowel movement every day?" her father asked.

"It's not necessary to have one every day," I said. "Some people have bowel movements three or four times a day, and some don't go for a week. Let Sally find a schedule that's good for her body. Don't train her to go to the bathroom like clockwork!"

Why, in human history, has it been so important to clean out your guts? Nobody ever got sick or died from irregular bowel movements now and then. But in the nineteenth century, especially, rich ladies and gentlemen rushed off to "health spas" to have their stools removed by enormous enemas, which were called "colonic irrigations." There are still resorts in this country—and more commonly in Europe—giving colonics to their patrons. Personally, I think a good laugh, or a round of tennis, is better for your guts and a lot less irritating.

I tell this to patients when I chat with them, and I do spend a lot of time chatting. The doctor-patient relationship has an immense impact on whether people get well, and stay well. Of course I can't talk away a cancer, or tell a patient with yellowed skin that the hepatitis I suspect will vanish if he just won't worry about it. But when patients are having gut reactions caused by emotional stress (and about 50 to 70 percent of my patients fall into this category), they need to know I understand and care about them and their pain. I'm not buddy-buddy with everyone, but I really like most of the people who come to my office. And they've somehow learned that talking to me makes them feel better. At the very least, I can reassure these patients that they don't have a dread disease.

Cardiologist Michael Halberstam once wrote "A doctor who enjoys holding hands with anxious patients is going to keep a lot of patients who need their hands held."

If a little hand-holding can change someone's life and make him happier and more productive, why not?

Many times, however, hand-holding won't help. That's what happened with eighteen-year-old Joanna, who came to me because she had persistent and chronic nausea and related vomiting for three years. "Food also sometimes sticks in my throat," she shrugged. "I don't know why."

Joanna was very pretty, but alarmingly thin. Her shiny platinum hair curled around bony shoulders and her rib cage jutted out like a stepladder. She was five feet five inches tall but weighed only ninety-three pounds. Despite this she told me she thought her major problem was being overweight.

When I heard that, I really got concerned. Some

youngsters, particularly girls, go on reckless diets, lost weight fast, and then can't seem to stop. It may turn into a psychological disease called *anorexia nervosa*. In severe cases patients suffer from malnutrition, getting thinner and thinner and all the time complaining about not being thin enough. Some of these girls starve themselves to death.

Joanna hadn't gone that far yet. I did blood counts and chemistry tests on her to rule out significant anemia or liver disease. X-rays showed that both her upper and lower guts were normal, and so were her endocrine studies. Joanna told me she'd seen two other doctors in the same year; I called them and they confirmed my feelings of no organic disease. She'd even had a complete workup at a major medical center and "all they told me to do was go see a psychiatrist," Joanna said glumly.

Joanna's school marks were excellent and she was a competitive, hard-driving teen-ager. She was also a "super athlete," but the nausea put a stop to her physical activities. She was afraid to go to college—where she'd already been accepted—because of the nausea and vomiting.

"There's nothing physically wrong with you, Joanna," I told her. "But there could be if you go on this way. You do need psychiatric help, and I recommend it, too."

Joanna looked at me. For a long time, she didn't speak. Then she said very slowly that she didn't see the need for a psychiatrist; she needed a good doctor. She also disagreed that she was too thin, and added, "I know what's best for my own body."

Patients like this are frustrating and difficult to

help because they seem hell-bent on self-destruction. Often, they come from families where one or both parents have some severe emotional disorders, but they refuse to see the connection. People like Joanna flit from doctor to doctor, and sometimes wind up having useless operations for phantom abdominal complaints.

In 1976 an extensive study was done at the Mayo Clinic by Dr. David W. Swanson, which suggested that the persistently nauseous patient might be committing some form of long-term suicide. The food-sticking and vomiting is part of the syndrome. It prevents the person from doing anything worthwhile in life, and together with the nausea results in abhorrence of food. Malnutrition and starvation follow unless the patient gets some competent long-term psychotherapy.

But you can't force someone to see a psychiatrist. They have to want to go, and Joanna was having none of it. Dr. Swanson said this type of behavior follows the pattern of most anorexia nervosa patients: they refuse significant psychiatric advice, maybe because they sense it's the only thing that will help. Since they are setting their own course for destruction, they don't want to be helped.

Joanna was like that. When she strode out of my office, I wondered, "How long before Joanna is dead?"

But there wasn't much time to brood about Joanna, because other patients were shuffling in the halls, or sitting naked in the examination rooms, or impatiently flipping the pages of worn magazines in my brown and blue waiting room.

Perhaps that's one blessing of being overworked as a doctor: you can't sit and pout about one patient. There are too many of them.

In one of the exam cubicles sat Marlo, a chubby, pleasant-looking twenty-four-year-old legal secretary. She smiled broadly at me when I came in, and seemed relaxed and cheerful. But her smile faded when she described her crippling symptoms: diarrhea and constipation, on and off, bloating and gas, and severe, wracking gut pain that kept her home from work and terrified her with thoughts of cancer or some other serious disease.

"I used to think it was a food allergy," Marlo explained, "because the pain was usually worse after I ate. I've seen several other doctors who told me to omit milk, but that didn't help, so I went back on it and there was no difference in my symptoms. Same with pizza, beans, coffee, and a bunch of other stuff. So, I just eat what I like." She patted her tummy. "Maybe too much," she added grimly. Then she smiled again. "I'm getting married soon, and it's been fun tasting the food we plan to have at the wedding reception. But, I'm really worried that I'll get these cramps during the ceremony. It would be awful . . ."

Marlo's voice trailed off. She looked sad for a moment, but soon brightened again, and I had no trouble getting her to tell me about her gut reactions.

Marlo had gut symptoms ever since high school. She was really a healthy young woman: no fever, chills, vomiting, blood in the stools or jaundice. But to make sure, I did a complete workup: X-rays, blood and stool studies, gallbladder tests, proctoscopy, and other tests. Everything seemed normal and the next time I saw Marlo—looking as cheerful as ever—I told her that she probably had an "irritable colon." That's another name for stress-caused gut symptoms.

Marlo was stunned. "But I'm so happy!" she exclaimed. "Why should I be having stomach-aches from stress?"

I told her that any exciting event, happy or unhappy, causes gut reactions in people who are prone to them. A delightful occurrence, such as getting married, can put a strain on you, even if it's the kind of strain you actively seek and enjoy. Gut reactors, by and large, are not passive people. They want things out of life, they work hard to get them, they plan and worry along the way, and they usually achieve their goals. Those are good traits in our society, and a lot of people—including me—act that way. But some gut reactors pay an unusual price. They may have to put up with a lot of pain at stressful points in their lives.

Marlo understood my explanation. She also confessed that she'd been on and off a lot of diets, such as high-carbohydrate, low-carbohydrate, high-protein, and so forth. I made her promise just to knock off sweets if she wanted to shed weight, and forget about those crazy diets. The same with the tranquilizers, aspirin, antacids, and other drugs that she pumped into her body now and then. I wanted to treat her with what I think is one of the best weapons against gut reactions: firm reassurance.

"First, you've had an excellent workup and I can tell you there is no organic disease," I told Marlo. "You're healthy."

"Second, there is no reason to believe you won't

stay healthy. Gut reactions don't lead to anything else. They may make you miserable at times, but gut symptoms caused by stress don't predispose a person to colitis, ulcers, cancer, or anything else. They won't protect you from these organic diseases, of course, but you have no greater chance of getting them than anybody else.

"Last, try to avoid frustrating or stressful events when you can. But don't let the symptoms interfere with your life. The pain may be bad, but it almost always goes away in a few minutes. I never heard of anyone with diarrhea so bad that they embarrassed themselves at their own wedding, so don't spend time scouting around for the nearest bathroom wherever you go. If you've got gas or bloating, take a brisk walk; sometimes that helps.

"The trick is," I told Marlo, "not to let gut reactions dominate your life. I know it isn't easy. But it's about all you can do right now, unless you decide to devote a lot of time and money to a psychiatrist."

When Marlo left, I thought about the immense amount of time and money, even excluding psychiatric care, that people spend on gut reactions. Dr. Albert I. Mendeloff of the Johns Hopkins University in Baltimore, Maryland, recently reported that in 1976 about 37,000 people in U.S. hospitals had "psychogenic gastrointestinal disorders." Another 96,000 patients were diagnosed as having "irritable bowel syndrome," which is the same thing. And another 85,000 people had one of these gut reaction syndromes listed as their secondary diagnosis; they had a disease, and also gut reactions.

It's my own hunch that most people with gut reactions never do land in the hospital, so when you add it up, there are immense numbers of people who suffer from stress-induced gastrointestinal malfunctions.

Dr. Mendeloff estimated that gut reactors spent 450,000 days a year in the hospital. So if you do some rough math on the problem, and multiply $300 per day (which is the average cost of a hospital stay) by 450,000 days, you come out with the staggering total of $135 million yearly being spent on hospital stays and evaluation tests on people with gut reactions. That doesn't take into account the money spent on drugstore potions or outpatient prescriptions, office visits, and lab tests, not to mention the money lost on sick days away from the office or on ruined vacations. So it costs the victims, in particular, and all of us in general, an enormous amount of money to cope with gut reactions. The pity of it all is that hospitalizations, drugs, and other usual remedies often are ineffective. What helps most is for the gut reactor to accept and learn to live with his affliction. And if it is any consolation, Dr. Mendeloff noted that of all the people who were hospitalized because of gut reactions, nobody died.

"I think I'm dying" was the first thing my next gut-reaction patient, Albert, said to me. He wasn't kidding. He was a forty-six-year-old college professor with heartburn so severe it woke him up at night, caused him to rush home from campus, and put a stop to his sex life.

Albert had no other symptoms. I did the usual exhaustive studies on him. Frankly, I thought they'd show some organic problem, because Albert's symptom was so specific, but he turned out to be in perfect health.

Albert's one really bad health habit of smoking two packs of cigarettes a day could make him a candidate for heart or lung disease, or possibly cancer of the esophagus. The esophagus is where his intense "heartburn" pain was coming from. So, when I ordered the usual lab tests, I included a cine-esophagram. Essentially, this test consists of a movie of the esophagus, and it did show a small hernia, or "popping out" of the esophagus. Still, that was a fairly common, minor problem. It wasn't enough to explain Albert's crippling pain. So I went further and inserted a long fiberoptic scope into his mouth and down into the esophagus, to have a first-hand look. Though this was uncomfortable for Albert, because he had to swallow a long rubber tube, it wasn't really painful. And, it's better than the old way doctors got their first-hand looks at a patient's insides, which was to do an "exploratory" operation. I took some pieces of tissue from Albert's esophagus, and lab tests confirmed my own sightings: normal.

Next, I did a Bernstein test, where acid is dripped into the esophagus to see if that brings on pain. It didn't. Albert showed a "negative Bernstein." Finally, I slid more tubes into Albert's esophagus to measure his swallowing pressure on a polygraph. This was the only test that turned out to be borderline; Albert had some increased spasms, or spikes, of swallowing waves, along with decreased tension of the lower esophageal sphincter. It got worse when Albert smoked a cigarette.

But still I wasn't satisfied. None of the results explained the horrible pain. By this time Albert was exhausted from the lab tests, worried, and anxious to talk. So, when I asked if his personal life was putting him under some stress, he said meekly, "I've been having an affair. It's over, but I feel guilty as hell. My wife and I have been married 18 years. We have two great kids, and the marriage is pretty good. I have no thoughts of leaving my wife, but I just wanted to get a little wild . . . have this affair . . . it was fun for a while.

"Now I don't know if I should tell my wife or not," Albert sighed. "The whole thing is making me feel . . . well . . . insecure. Suppose she gets really mad, and wants to leave?"

It didn't take much to convince Albert that telling his wife was better than wondering, and being in intolerable pain. Of course, I couldn't run his emotional life for him. But I could make suggestions, offer understanding and sympathy, and prescribe a few medical rules: First, I told Albert, *don't smoke;* don't eat before bedtime, because eating and then lying down flat can cause "reflux," or a spitting up of gastric juices; cut down on coffee and fruit juices because they have a high acid content; eliminate aspirin; sleep with the head of the bed elevated about six to nine inches. A lot of pillows under your head won't help. The whole bed needs to be tilted so gravity will prevent reflux; and don't take anti-spasmodic drugs because they often slow down the food-emptying process and make the heartburn worse. There is one new drug that sometimes helps. It's called cimetidine. It stops the body's frenzied manufacturing of gastric acid. One cimetidine a night, plus the other measures I prescribed, helped Albert feel considerably better. A few weeks later he called to tell me that the heartburn had all but gone away. He added that the pain really began to fade the night he told his wife about his "fling," as he put it, and she said she understood, and still loved him.

Your spouse and your family are an important influence on the way your guts behave. Too often, patients tell me what they can't or won't tell the person with whom they've lived for ten or twenty years. They can't communicate so their unruly stomachs scream for them. On the outside, gut reactors may be quiet, even placid people. Inside, they're in turmoil.

That's the way it was with the last gut reactor I'll describe, Alexia. She was a fifty-eight-year-old waitress whose abdominal pains were so severe that she could barely stand up in my examining room.

Alexia was divorced. She was also a grand-mother. Her pain had been present for five months, and she described it as being "just above my belly button, and there all the time, sometimes worse than others."

The pain was driving her mad, Alexia said. She drank and smoked a lot because of it. She missed days from her job because of it too, and her boss was threatening to fire her. She was nibbling junk food out of nervousness, and had gained ten pounds since the pain started.

Weight gain is not usually a sign of disease; in fact, it's often just the opposite so I was a little relieved when Alexia told me about it. She went on talking in a bland, low monotone, exhibiting the depression I've come to associate with older gut reactors. Life was over for her, Alexia sighed. She couldn't sleep, she had no energy, and she had neck and back trouble and headaches in addition to her gut pain.

When Alexia was in her 30's, at the time of her first divorce, she had a nervous breakdown. She also had two husbands, and both of them were alcoholics. They left her with four children, and Alexia now had six grandchildren. She took care of them from time to time and once enjoyed it, she said, but now "I'm just losing interest in them."

Clearly, one of Alexia's main problems was unhappiness, but I couldn't rule out organic disease yet. She did have a troublesome medical history of multiple operations, including a hysterectomy and gallbladder removal. When I examined Alexia she seemed in good physical shape: there were no swollen glands in her neck or armpits; her heart and lungs sounded normal; there were no masses, tenderness, or enlargement in her abdomen; bowel sounds were normal; and the lymph nodes in the groin were not enlarged. My major impression of this sad, teary-eyed lady was that life held no joy for her, and her guts were reacting with despair.

But I couldn't be sure. As with every other case of suspected gut reactions, it's important to put the patient through as many diagnostic tests as needed to be able to say, "I'm reasonably certain we can rule out organic disease."

Alexia's pains had gone on for a long time, and they were centered in one spot, which could be a sign of trouble. I checked for liver disease, did urine and stool studies, and looked for a metabolic disease such as thyroid or diabetes. Everything was normal. When the X-rays revealed that Alexia's upper and lower GI (gastrointestinal) tract and kidneys were normal, I went further with an intravenous cholangiogram. This is a sophisticated X-ray of the bile ducts, but since Alexia's gallbladder was gone, the X-rays didn't come out well. I had trouble reading them, so I insisted on two more sophisticated tests. One was an ultrasound reading of the abdomen, which painlessly bounces sound waves off the pancreas and liver and outlines them on a graph. Another is the CT scan, which is another exacting X-ray procedure. CT is short for "computerized tomography." It often does better than other X-rays in pinpointing the smallest flaw in a patient's organs.

There were no flaws in Alexia's organs. Still she was hurting, and at her age pain can come from some well-hidden sources. So I asked her to go into the hospital for seven or eight days for observation and more tests. Most people groan at this, disagree with me, or get scared. Some even smile and say, "That'll be a nice vacation," and then go off and cry their eyes out. Alexia didn't react at all. I had the feeling her emotions had turned her to jelly.

While Alexia was in the hospital, I asked a psychologist to see her. Sure enough, he reported "a marked degree of depression and feelings of frustration and ineffectualness, with a degree of anger being apparently suppressed on the surface." Her physical workup was normal.

To me, Alexia was a classic example of a problem in an older age group. It gives both patients and their doctors a lot of trouble. The doctors call it "cryptic abdominal pain that defies diagnosis." Patients call it "stomach gas and pain." I call it gut reactions.

Psychological depression caused changes in Alexia's gut, which in turn resulted in pain. And like so many older people, I'm afraid she'll never get rid of all of it. She's had a hard, up-and-down life, and although she's a bright woman, she never acquired the skills to help her get a decent job. I've said that gut reactors are "driven" people, but Alexia's drive, apparently, was in a self-destructive direction. She also had some other destructive tendencies: she hurt herself by marrying unstable men, putting up with a demanding, unfriendly boss, and even agreeing to care for grandchildren on weekends when she should be having fun with people her own age.

I started Alexia on a round of antidepressants, and gave her as much reassurance as I could. I warned her not to take tranquilizers, sedatives, sleeping pills, or alcohol. They're all depressants. I told her again and again her pain was the result of a deep psychological need—her body's way of calling for emotional help—and I recommended a good psychiatrist. She said she'd see him but when she left I had the feeling that Alexia didn't believe my diagnosis.

It's easy to understand her skepticism. Most people, when they hit fifty or so, are terrified of pain in the gut, especially because it could signal cancer. We all know some cancers are difficult to diagnose in the early stages. Other tumors can cause persistent gut pain that also defies diagnosis, and just because routine tests come out normal, the doctor can't be sure he hasn't missed something. But when sophisticated tests also are negative, when the patient's every action and word seem to confirm your hunch about emotional problems, and especially when the pain goes on for a long time without changing, you can be reasonably sure it's gut reactions. Organic pain just doesn't go on and on; a disease changes, grows, usually gets worse. Gut reactions, for the most part, stay the same.

Not every doctor believes such intense pain can come from emotional sources. I know perfectly fine physicians who see an older patient with stubborn pain, grow impatient with the "normal" findings on the tests, and do an abdominal "exploratory" operation. I'll say flatly that these operations are a bad mistake. They're expensive, painful, and dangerous, and rarely do doctors find a thing.

It is frustrating to encounter a patient with alarming symptoms, put him or her through batteries of expensive and undignified—and sometimes painful—tests, and then find nothing. But I tell all the people I know with gut reactions *not* to rely heavily on a medical cure. Good medicine can help manage gut symptoms, but a cure can only come from an alteration in the way you react to life's stresses.

Since all of us are constantly battered by stress, many patients ask why they, and not all of us, have gut reactions. I don't know the answer, and to my knowledge neither does anyone else. Perhaps some people are born with an organic predetermination to gut distress. And it makes sense to assume that if your family, friends, or social group puts a lot of emphasis on food and digestion, you'll grow up with a heightened awareness of the gastrointestinal process. Still, there are no firm answers about gut reactions. The best you can do now to prevent needless worry is to use the information in the next chapter, which describes what goes on in your body when you're having gut reactions.

2

Looking Inside

So your guts are giving you trouble.

You are not alone. Many people who pile into doctors' offices are having the same symptoms: gas, bloating, constipation, diarrhea, vomiting, stomach churning, heartburn, difficulty in swallowing, and wrenching pain.

Most of these people are not dangerously sick. They are upset. Their boiling emotions are causing malfunction of the digestive system. They are having gut reactions.

It's normal, in our hectic world, to get upset. Stress is part of modern life. But when stress becomes internalized, and causes gut reactions, it's time to fight back. It's time to bring your troubled digestive system under control.

You *can* do it. And the best way to start is by understanding the structure and function of your own gastrointestinal tract. Once you know what your guts look like and what functions they perform, you'll realize how emotions can easily turn over your inner applecart.

There are a lot of feelings associated with your guts. Hunger, fullness, passing gas, or wishing to move your bowels are all normal feelings coming from the digestive system. But there is a thin line between those normal feelings and the "abnormal" symptoms you get when the system has gone awry. The gastrointestinal tract is huge, and takes up a lot of space inside your body; stretched out, your intestines would be about thirty feet long. But this long tube, which acts like a subway system for the transportation of food through the body, is curled and looped around other organs. Because it is so big, and packed pretty tightly inside you, it is hard to tell when the annoyance of a little gas bubble turns into real discomfort, or when a bellyache escalates into crippling pain.

When that happens, however, a lot of anxiety can be erased if you know where the annoyance or pain is coming from.

Trouble can start the instant you touch food to your lips and it comes in contact with the soft lining inside your mouth. This is where the intestinal tract starts, too. Salivary glands are in your mouth. They secrete the sticky liquid—saliva— which contains the enzymes to begin the digestion of food. As soon as your teeth and jaws start churning, breaking the food into small pieces so it can be swallowed, saliva squirts into your mouth. Some doctors have said this secretion is so potent it could dissolve almost anything you choose to eat.

Soon you have a sticky mass of saliva and crushed food that must be swallowed. Swallowing is an active movement of muscles; its purpose is to push food from the mouth to the esophagus, without letting the food get into the "windpipe," or trachea. If your reflexes, nerves, and muscles are undisturbed while you attempt to swallow, the food will pass normally to the back of your "food pipe," or pharynx. At the same time the muscles of the windpipe automatically close. But if stress is present, either at the moment you are swallowing or if it is lurking in your subconscious all the time, that delicate swallowing mechanism can be disturbed. The muscles may tighten, causing you to gag. Or there might be a reverse peristalsis, or backward movement of the muscles, which will cause you to vomit.

No wonder, when people are confronted with bad news, they might exclaim, "I can't swallow that!" Or, if they are disgusted with a friend's behavior, they could declare that "You make me vomit."

Once food gets from the mouth to the esophagus, muscle activity picks up a lot. The esophagus is a long tube which propels food into your stomach. Muscles ripple along this tube in little rhythmic waves. If the rhythm is disturbed—most often by stress—you will feel some blockage in your throat, and food will be hard to swallow. A terrified college student, getting ready to take oral exams, might tell his doctor "I'm sweating and I can't get my food down. It feels like something is sticking in my throat." This is called *dysphagia* or *globus*. Both of these words simply mean the muscles pushing food into your stomach are upset. This can happen when a tumor or some other physical blockage is present. But much of the time it is muscle tension caused by stress.

At the end of the esophagus is the lower esophageal sphincter. It is like the screw-on cap at the end of the tube. If the sphincter does not work properly—if it is not tight enough—it will allow partly digested food to leak back up into the esophagus. The result? You get heartburn.

Heartburn has nothing to do with your heart. You just feel the burning sensation in your upper chest, where most people assume the heart is located. The "burn" comes from the strong digestive juices that, when they get into the wrong place, instantly irritate the lining of the esophagus. Disease can loosen the esophageal valve. So can too much alcohol or spicy foods. The resulting acid "burn" can turn into irritation or ulceration of the esophagus. But most often the problem is stress, which causes the sphincter to malfunction. The "burn" either can be relieved with drugstore tablets, or it goes away by itself.

Heartburn may be a continual problem with people who eat under stressful conditions. One young mother, who told me she could never complete a meal at home without feeling "that awful burning sensation," felt much better when she stopped trying to discipline her rowdy youngsters at the dinner table. She decided to feed them first, then sat down later to a quiet meal with her husband. The mealtime stress went away, and so did her heartburn.

Once food is safely past the esophagus, and the esophageal sphincter, it goes into the stomach. This important organ serves three life-giving functions: it churns up food, adds chemicals to break the food down, and passes this nourishment plus waste materials further along the digestive pipeline. The stomach is so important, in fact, that any time you have a disturbance anywhere along the digestive tract you are likely to complain of an "upset stomach" even if the distress does not originate from the stomach at all. And the stomach is a recognized center for emotional turmoil. Why else would you say, "I can't stomach that," or "You make me sick to my stomach."

The stomach is a big, pulpy, balloonlike organ located just below the spot where the two sides of your rib cage come together. It is about fifteen or twenty inches long and can expand to hold several quarts of food and liquid. When it is healthy, a doctor can look into your stomach with a long, flexible, see-through tube, and spot a rosy, smooth stomach lining. A diseased stomach will be dark red and bumpy. If you have been complaining of stomach pain or other gut disorders, and chemical tests show no signs of disease, a doctor who is specially trained in the procedure might look directly into your stomach with this tube, called a gastroesophagoscope. This procedure—which is only mildly uncomfortable, because you have to swallow the tube—often eliminates the need for exploratory surgery. Surgery of the stomach can cause lifelong problems if it damages this delicate organ. The stomach needs to be in prime condition to secrete hydrochloric acid and pepsin, which breaks down the protein in meat and other foods. A damaged stomach often cannot function properly.

Action is always going on in the digestive tract, and the stomach is a prime place where all the normal jiggling, crushing, and churning movements of your inner body get out of control. If you pump too much food into the stomach too fast, irritate it with drugs or alcohol, or allow stress to over-stimulate it, your stomach is likely to give you a lot of pain.

If you're undergoing mild stress, you probably won't double over with pain; the most you'll suffer is the familiar "butterflies in the stomach." Every actor gets this queasy feeling before he steps on stage. The "butterflies" are mild digestive tract muscular spasms, caused by anxiety, tension, or stress. They usually go away when you become absorbed in an interesting activity. An actor's "butterflies" generally flutter away during Act I.

From the stomach, food moves on to the small intestine. A valve at the end of the stomach, called the *pyloric sphincter*, closes off and keeps the food from coming back from the small intestine into the stomach again. By this time, food is pretty well loaded with normal body chemicals, and ready to be absorbed into the bloodstream so its nutrients can be transported to all your throbbing, hungry organs.

But first, the food passes into the upper part of the small intestine, the duodenum. The bile duct is located here. This duct empties secretions from the liver, gallbladder, and pancreas into the duodenum. These secretions all help in the further breakdown of the food.

The liver contributes yellow-green bile. Without a liver, life would end. This squishy red organ secretes enzymes and hormones to keep your body moving. It also acts as your personal "detoxification system" by getting rid of foreign materials like alcohol or drugs that you might pump into your body.

Another important organ that juts off the small intestine is the pancreas, which adds amylase, lipase, and other enzymes to the digestive process. In addition to aiding digestion, the pancreas produces insulin, a chemical necessary to metabolize sugar in the body. You can live without a pancreas, although you would be diabetic and would need injections of insulin and other enzymes to keep going.

The gallbladder is next. The juices that pour out of the gallbladder have already been secreted by the liver. They are also part of the way we talk about stress when we say "He galls me," or "You've got your gall!" When the stress is overwhelming, and perhaps too much of these fiery liquids mix in the digestive system, the result may be pain in the small intestine and other symptoms of a gut reaction.

The gallbladder's sole function is to store the bile which is constantly being made by the liver. You do not need all that bile all the time, so nature has provided a place to store it. If you get gallstones, it means that the function of this storage house has been disturbed and the bile has become lumpy. This can lead to infection and the possible surgical removal of the gallbladder. That's okay; you don't need the gallbladder. Your body will naturally handle the bile flow.

The small intestine has two other parts, in addition to the duodenum. The second part is called the *jejunum;* it is simply the middle part of this long coil. The end part is called the *ileum.* This leads into the *cecum*, which is the first part of the large intestine. The function of all of these parts is the same: food absorption. All along the way, enzymes are attacking the food and breaking it down.

The appendix, a useless organ, hangs like a little limp balloon from the cecum. When you get appendicitis, you have an infection of this annoying organ, which one doctor exclaimed is in the body "to aggravate parents, hurt people, and give surgeons some business."

During the time the food is being pushed along the digestive tract, there is some movement of nourishment into the body. But most of the vitamins, fats, carbohydrates, and proteins we need to get from food are squeezed out of it in the small intestines. The intestinal wall has many pores; these are in tiny fingerlike projectiles called *villi*. The villi filter the food, now turned into liquid, into the bloodstream, so it can be carried to the waiting body cells.

Now, most of what is left is waste material, which must be dumped outside the body. As it gets moved from the small intestine (which is called "small" only because it is skinny) into the large intestine (which is short and fat), about ninety-five percent of the "food" is already used up. In the colon the water, nonabsorbable food particles, and bacteria become semisolid fecal material. It leaves the body through the rectum and the cycle is complete.

But trouble may not end there. *Hemorrhoids*, which are little blood vessels at the end of the rectal canal, may act up. Everyone has hemorrhoids. But when they get inflamed or infected, the blood vessels become engorged, and they hurt. Then, you have *thrombosed hemorrhoids*. That interferes with easy bowel movement, and can lead to gut problems all along the line.

It works the other way, too. If you have gut reactions somewhere in your digestive tract, you'll probably have irregular or difficult bowel movements. You'll strain, and the straining can cause inflamed hemorrhoids. Thus, this painful swelling in your rectum is often a result of stress. When you spot some annoying person pushing his way toward you at a party, and you try to avoid him because he's "a pain in the ass," you're referring to the stress factor in swollen hemorrhoids.

The whole digestive process, when it is normal, takes from twelve to twenty-four hours. When things go smoothly—when stress or disease does not interfere—you hardly feel the frenzied activity that is going on inside your body. But when you tense up, causing the various muscles involved to contract or to go into spasm, you can become agonizingly aware of every little inner movement.

That awareness, most often felt as pain somewhere in the gut, is not illness. It is a disruption in the function of the digestive system; literally, an "upset." If you emerge from a troublesome situation, get away from the person who is annoying you, or even let out the tension with a stream of curses, the "upset" goes away, and so does the pain.

Because the digestive tract is so complex, pain or distress can come from almost any point in its jungle of muscle, nerve endings, blood vessels, and secretory cells. The tract is crisscrossed with thin, hairlike blood vessels which bring in oxygen and take out food that has been absorbed. White blood cells, lymph glands, and tissue cells also infiltrate the lining of the tract and can be disturbed by shock, disease, disgust or overactive emotions. The very important "chief cells" located in the stomach may be microscopic, but they, perhaps, can cause a giant-sized bellyache if they react to stress and oversecrete the hydrochloric acid you need to digest your meat. Special "antral" cells are also located in the stomach at its lower end, the antrum. They secrete a hormone, called *gastrin*, which stimulates the chief cells. So an upset in one tiny part of the digestive tract may set off a chain reaction that can have you squirming with a belly-ache for hours.

Being upset can also cause you to gasp or gulp air. Then you will get gas. Gas from above is called belching, and from below it is called *flatus*. Gas also can be manufactured in the digestive tract, when things go haywire and the tract becomes overactive. An increase in mucous, which passes through the rectum, is also brought on by digestive overactivity. So is a sudden spurt, or sudden decrease, of saliva in your mouth. That's why shock, sudden anger, or even mild tension often gives you a dry mouth. Why else would public speakers always need a pitcher of water near them on the podium? They're nervous, and they need the water because their mouths are dry.

These are all gut reactions. They are the way your digestive system signals it is being affected by your emotions. In every case, the symptoms—the gut reactions—are *real*. You do not imagine the pain, gas, mucous, or dry mouth. They are hap-pening because your body is making a physical response to an emotional cause.

Most of the time, these physical responses are completely normal, even if they are annoying or painful. All of us, from time to time, burp, pass gas, feel bloated, lose all appetite, get nauseated, have heartburn, or struggle with diarrhea or constipation. Even an occasional sharp pain is part of the complicated digestive process. It is when the symptom pops up again and again, and interferes with your work, play, or homelife, that it becomes a medical problem.

More often than not, these gut symptoms are *functional*. This means that although the *functions* of the digestive system are being interrupted or upset somewhere along the way, no identifiable organic disease is present. A *function* is going wrong. You're upset, but you are not sick. You're having a gut reaction.

Your guts will also react, somewhat more severely, to disease. It's important to know the basic differences between gut reactions caused by emotional upset and gut problems caused by disease. An emotional gut reaction hurts, but it won't kill you. It can wait. But a gut disease needs swift medical attention.

A major sign of a digestive disease is bleeding. When you pass blood from the rectum, pass black or tarlike stools, or vomit up blood, your body is calling for help . . . fast. Consistent loss of weight (when you are not on a diet); severe, lasting pain; fever; or jaundice, which is a yellowing of the skin or the whites of your eyes, always calls for an immediate trip to the doctor.

Sometimes, your digestive tract will be unable to absorb food properly, and you will be plagued with diarrhea, or fatty, foul-smelling stools. This could signal liver, pancreatic, or gallbladder disease. This needs a doctor's care. Perhaps some of the chugging chemical factories in your small intestine aren't pumping out the right secretions, or enough of them. Infection or tumor could be the cause, not emotional distress.

Some people are born with a blockage in the intestinal tract, or abnormally formed liver ducts, or shortened intestines. Usually, these congenital defects can be remedied, but they could cause mild digestive problems throughout life. These problems can get much worse when the person is emotionally upset.

Infections also cause symptoms that can be mistaken for gut reactions. Viruses can cause gastroenteritis and its accompanying gas, pain, and digestive tract irritability. Hepatitis, a liver disease that makes you weak for months, is caused by a virus. So is the painful *pancreatitis*, an inflammation of the pancreas. Parasites and certain bacteria can invade the digestive tract, and turn your inner world upside down with everything from vomiting to diarrhea. Inflammation, ulcers, blood vessel diseases, cancer, mixed-up metabolism, and the simple eating of spoiled or heavily spiced foods all can produce fake gut reactions. They are "fake" only because these problems are not coming from an emotional cause. They will show up in tests or on X-rays and the doctor can usually make a quick diagnosis. They are *organic*, but not *functional*, problems.

It is only when reasonable tests show up negative, and X-rays all look "normal," that you could be a victim of functional disease, or gut reactions. The gut reactions take longer to diagnose and they often frustrate both you und your doctor because they have no apparent cause. It may take a long time, and some soul-searching, before you begin to connect your spiteful boss with the stomach cramp you get when you walk into the office.

But don't let anyone tell you the discomfort of a gut reaction is "all in your head." It's not! You feel pain or discomfort because something is actually happening in your digestive system. Usually a muscle is going into spasm, or an acid secretion is spilling into the wrong organ. Something physical is happening inside you when you have a gut reaction. That "something," however, is not caused by organic disease. It is caused by emotion.

"When this happens, I say a patient is having subjective symptoms without objective findings," said one gastric specialist. "Most of the time, a gut reaction is harmless, and can be brought under control if the patient understands what is going on."

Now that you have a better idea of what is "going on" inside your digestive tract, you are ready to learn the major differences between gut distress and gut disease.

3

Distress or Disease?

It's important for many reasons to know the differences between the symptoms of serious organic disease and a nervous, unruly intestinal tract due to stress. It can help you decide whether to dash to the doctor immediately or to self-medicate and watch for a while. It can ease the worry you might feel about your illness, a worry that will add to the stress and just make your symptoms worse. And it can convince you to stop dwelling on organic disease, accept the final diagnosis of gut reactions, and start making the changes necessary to bring you relief.

There is a way to be reasonably sure your pain is a gut reaction: time. Symptoms that last only a few days, or even a week, and then go away, are probably not a sign of serious disease. Doctors call this a "self-limited" symptom. This test of time also applies to a symptom that has been with you for a long time without any change or progression. If you've been feeling gut pain, nausea, or other symptoms for over six months or a year, and your doctor can't find anything wrong with you, your problem is probably functional, not organic.

Time isn't the only way to tell the difference between gut disease and gut reactions. One common-sense question you can ask yourself is, "How do I feel?" If you are in pain, but still feel peppy enough to jog around the block and your appetite is good, you're probably not sick. Still, you won't be satisfied until the third and most important measurement is applied: *objective findings*.

An objective finding is a body change that you yourself can see, or that your doctor can record or find by an examination or a lab test. Are you noticing an involuntary weight loss? Is there any yellow discoloration of your skin or the whites of your eyes? The yellowness usually indicates jaundice, and both it and the weight loss cannot be denied; they are not gut reactions. Maybe only your doctor, on examination, can make an objective finding of a swollen, enlarged gland or lymph node, or a large, tender liver. These also are indicative of organic, not stress-induced, trouble. Another type of objective finding that only your doctor can make comes from a lab test. These tests are really an extension of the physician's hands, eyes, and ears. For instance, a blood test can show an objective finding of anemia or low-blood count. It could show abnormal liver function. Another objective finding is an X-ray clearly showing an ulcer or a tumor.

In addition to how you feel and objective findings, another way to get at the differences between disease and distress is to take a look at what is happening in your life at the time you experience your symptoms. Are you in the middle of another real illness or body malfunction—even a broken leg—that's upsetting you? Are you indulging in alcohol, taking drugs, or even overdoing some prescribed medications? Have you changed your job, moved to a new neighborhood, altered your diet, or taken a big trip? All of these things can throw your digestive system into turmoil and cause gut reactions.

Even if you can pinpoint your distress enough to suspect either real disease or gut reactions, it's not easy to be sure. That's especially true if you use the first barometer I suggested: feeling good, or not. You can feel weak and tired, have difficulty working or concentrating, lose interest in play or sex, or even have a hard time getting along with family or friends. All of this comes out as "just not feeling good." It is such a common symptom, historically, that the main word in illness comes from this feeling: "dis-ease," which is simply defined as the state of not being at ease. Physicians use the terms "mal-ease" or "malaise" or "poor ease" or "bad ease."

This feeling can be related to almost any significant organic disease, or it can be related to tension, stress, or psychiatric problems. Don't expect to take this symptom alone and come to any significant conclusion. If not feeling good persists over a few days, and if it affects your life-style, go to a physician. It's his or her job to relate your "poor ease" to some real "dis-ease."

Even loss of appetite, and resulting loss of weight, can be due to physical or emotional factors. Systemic symptoms such as "bloating" or "gas" also are too generalized to make you feel sure about whether or not you are really sick. Again, if the symptoms are short-lived, they probably should not be taken too seriously. Also, if these symptoms were present in the past, and past checkups have not revealed disease, then they, too, can be felt to be part of an emotional or stress reaction.

One symptom that is definitely *not* a stress reaction is fever. Almost always, a rise in your body temperature that persists more than a day means infection or disease; it calls for a trip to your doctor. If you throw up blood, this could mean gastrointestinal bleeding. Immediately report it to your doctor. Passing blood in the stools, or black, tarry stools indicating a breakdown of red blood by bacteria to black, iron-containing material, requires a doctor's immediate attention. If there is marked abdominal distention (swelling) with pain, you should go to your doctor. And, again, if your skin or eyes are yellow, that's a pretty objective and important indication of liver disease.

Objective findings should never be ignored. However, it is not unknown for some very upset people to show blood, swelling, or even a change in skin color as a result of stress. One Atlanta psychiatrist reported having a patient "pee blood" out of fear of getting on an airplane. The patient's father, it was discovered, also had blood in his urine when he got very scared about taking a plane trip. So, how can you rely on these so-called objective symptoms to tell if you are sick?

You can't. You can just use them as one additional tool to help in your diagnosis. They should bring you to your doctor, who will have to use his own physical exams, plus lab tests, to come up with more objective signs of specific disease.

Lab tests are usually the last word in determining the difference between gut disease and gut reactions. If X-rays, blood tests, scans, or ultrasound "bounces" show no disease, it's time to question your mental state. Are you depressed, anxious, or going through external distress such as a divorce or a job change? Are you just having some overall anxiety for no known reason? (The reason *is* known, but only in your subconscious. You won't find that reason without a psychiatrist's help.) All this means your problem is probably functional. Let your doctor help you find out for sure.

So, you have taken your ill body, with its symptoms, to a doctor. You have gone through all the required lab tests. No organicity or disease shows up, but you still feel gut symptoms.

What now?

Should you forget about it? Should you keep seeing the physician you are seeing? Should you consult another physician for a second opinion? Or should you look for some organized means of psychotherapy such as a psychiatrist, psychologist, or group treatment?

These are very important questions at this point in your life. The answers will be different for each person, because some people are more concerned about their symptoms, or have a more phobic reaction towards the possibility of a major disease than others. Here are your alternatives:

It is your *perception* of symptoms that may be your guide for further medical intervention. People with a great deal of insight into their own behavior may find it easy to decide which route to follow after a thorough gastroenterological evaluation. But I would say most people do not have that insight. So, what you do next depends on how you perceive, or how you "see," your troubled tummy.

Are you reassured that there is no physical disease? Then you are probably responding to the authority of the gastroenterologist. You are impressed by the time and attention of your physician and the complicated diagnostic tests that have been done. You accept the final diagnosis that your tummy troubles are functional and there is no organic base. If so, you do not need further medical intervention. Try to forget the problem, and go about your business. If you force yourself to do it, your body will probably react by giving up the symptoms and the trouble will go away by itself.

But suppose that in spite of your doctor's reassurances, you remain tense and nervous. You feel some skepticism. You think much more can be done, and you're not totally convinced that one doctor is the "court of last resort." You want another opinion, and possibly more tests. Then you should *have* another opinion! Contact a consulting gastroenterologist or go through a major national diagnostic center such as the Mayo Clinic or other medical school or referral center. But I will be honest: You may wind up back with your first doctor for follow-up care. It may take years of doctor-hopping for you to finally accept the gut reaction diagnosis. Only then will you need no further complicated active medical intervention.

Suppose your symptoms, to you, are crippling?

If you can't go on with your personal or business life because of constant gut pain or other uncomfortable bodily reactions, you probably need psychiatric care. This doesn't mean you are crazy. In fact, just the opposite is true; you are sane enough—and brave enough—to know you need help. And instead of complaining and staying a cripple, you are going to go and *get that help*.

Before you do go, however, you may experience what doctors call "symptom shifting." Your gastrointestinal symptoms may go away and be replaced with other problems, such as headache, chest pain, or other bad feelings. This may tempt you to see other specialists, who will then attempt to find an organic cause for the new symptoms. This could go on forever, so it is best to recognize that symptom shifting is your body's way of trying to find a non-psychological cause for your pain. Force yourself to stay away from new doctors, and admit you need psychological or psychiatric consultation and treatment.

Essentially, my recommendations of what you can do now are based on how you accept your doctor's findings that you have gut reactions, and not disease. The recommendations are also based on your perception of how severe the symptoms may be. Dr. Arthur J. Barsky III, of the Department of Psychiatry of the Massachusetts General Hospital, reported in an article in the *Annals of Internal Medicine* in 1979 that there is a great variety in the way patients respond to symptoms. In the article, called "Patients Who Amplify Bodily Sensations," Dr. Barsky states that psychological, sociocultural, or even medical factors all contribute to the way a patient views his pain or other gut symptoms. One patient can have intense alarm, worry, and disability, and even a reluctance to relinquish these symptoms because they serve some internal need; they may be an attention-getting device, for example. The opposite is the patient who actually minimizes, ignores, or represses his symptoms. These patients tend to deny their illness. But many patients get what Dr. Barsky calls "secondary gain" from symptoms, and this tends to amplify their response. There are three kinds of secondary gains, says Dr. Barsky: "Number One is sympathy, attention, and support, including financial support. Number Two is being excused from various duties, responsibilities, obligations or challenges. Number Three is the ability to manipulate and influence important people by virtue of their acceptance of the individual as being sick."

These secondary gains can't be easily recognized by a nonpsychiatrist. You, as a patient, may not even realize them yourself. It's hard to admit to yourself that the searing pain you get after dinner is a way to force your spouse into doing the dishes. In any case, you'd need a mental health expert to help you recognize what is going on in your body, and how it relates to what is going on in your mind.

Society sometimes encourages an amplification of gut symptoms. We're now living in an era of great concern about health. Dr. Robert H. Moser, Executive Vice-President of the American College of Physicians, published an essay in September, 1979, in *Forum on Medicine*, called "The Prognosis of the Species." Dr. Moser's point in this article was that our society is so concerned about all the various things affecting our health that we live with tremendous concern "something bad" is going to happen to our bodies. Although Americans seem to be relatively healthy, and have a reasonably long life-span, we all worry about food additives, environmental influences, nuclear reactions, cigarettes, inactivity, overweight, underweight, and the undocumented claims that vitamins, special diets, and exercise can either prolong our lives—or end them abruptly. Dr. Moser says, "The new danger to our well-being, if we continue to listen to all the talk, is becoming a nation of healthy hypochondriacs, living gingerly and worrying ourselves half to death."

Some people will worry more than others. Dr. Douglas A. Drossman, of the University of North Carolina, summarized three factors which make a person worry about health in an article on the "Irritable Bowel Syndrome," published in the *Journal of Gastroenterology* in 1977. First, he said, some people simply have a psychological predisposition to health worries. Dr. Drossman gives the example of the child who is observed getting gratification from defecation. The child then learns that bowel control is rewarded by praise, and that soiling will lead to punishment and rejection. He therefore develops, through the use of the bowel, various degrees of self-assertiveness, compliance, or even obstinacy. When he grows older, he continues to use some of these same bowel habits to control others. That person will value his control, and worry about his body a lot.

The second factor that makes a person a worrier could be an organic weakness centering on the gastrointestinal tract. A person who is born with a "weak" tract will make it a target organ for his or her emotional problems. The lack of knowledge in this area is overwhelming.

If you add a third factor—what Dr. Drossman calls an "environmental stress factor"—you can understand a third reason why some people worry about their bodies more than others. The environmental stress factor is a change in life-style or role that upsets you. It will signal the onset of functional illness in most susceptible people.

These factors exist in all people to some extent, and are most severe in patients with functional disease of the GI tract. Dr. Steven J. Young, a psychiatrist in Kalamazoo, Michigan, reported on this in an article called "Psychiatric Consideration in Irritable Bowel Syndrome." The article was published in *The Journal of Practical Gastroenterology* in July and August, 1979. Dr. Young looked at people with gut pain and found that in twenty percent there was hysteria, twenty-two percent were depressed, eleven percent had anxiety, only one percent were alcoholics, and twenty-three percent had an undiagnosed psychiatric illness. This came to a whopping seventy-seven percent of patients with irritable bowel who had significant psychiatric problems. Dr. Young's study may lead to an overemphasis on the significance of psychiatric diseases in functional GI tract problems, because only the sickest patients go to psychiatric centers where they get into studies like this. However, his study does point up evidence of anxiety or depression in a lot of people with functional GI disease.

How can you tell if you are anxious or depressed? You need to be in what Dr. Young calls a "dysphoric mood." That means you feel depressed, sad, irritable, or worried. And you need at least four of the following symptoms: 1) Poor appetite with weight loss of at least two pounds in a week or ten pounds in a year without dieting; 2) Insomnia or hypersomnia, which is sleeping too little or too much; 3) Fatigue, or loss of energy; 4) Difficulty in moving around or unusual clumsiness, shaking, or hyperactive movements; 5) Decreased interest in your usual activities, or diminished sexual drive; 6) Feelings of self-reproach or guilt; 7) Impaired thinking or concentration; 8) Recurrent thoughts of death or suicide.

Besides anxiety and depression, hysteria is common in people with gut reactions. This usually begins in young people, and doctors say hysteria is determined by at least twenty medically unexplained symptoms. Generally speaking, hysterical people usually have a history of undergoing hospitalization and surgical procedures. Put simply, these are patients with chronic medical illnesses of various types. Frequently they become drug abusers, because so much medication is prescribed for them by doctors.

By now, you've probably seen yourself described in a variety of ways. And by now you should have a deeper understanding of the differences between gut distress and gut disease. Together, you and your doctor can decide what comes next. Right now your main task—discussed in the next chapter—is finding the doctor who is right for you.

4

The Right Doctor

I'm amazed at the way people pick their doctors.
Women get my name from their hairdressers or
neighbors; men come to me on a bartender's
advice. People in pain pluck my name from the
telephone book; one sweet schoolteacher told me,
"You sounded like you had a 'smart' name."
Most patients come because my office is close to
their homes or jobs, or my secretary found an
appointment time convenient for them. So they
come, for these frivolous reasons, and place their
bodies and lives in my hands.

Sometimes I grit my teeth when I think that for
many people, picking a doctor takes second place
to picking a car mechanic. I know folks who
agonize longer about which restaurant will get
their Saturday-night business than which doctor
will get to work on their guts.

How *should* you select your gastroenterologist?
Ideally, he or she will be recommended by your

family physician. Sometimes the same friendly face you've been seeing for years—your family "doc"—will be able to treat your stomachache. But if it goes much further than an ache, "doc" will turn you over to someone like me: a specially educated, specially trained, and specially equipped gastroenterologist. I'm always pleased when another doctor calls or writes and says, "I want you to see my patient." It's a pat on the back, because it says, "I trust you. You know what you're doing, and most of your patients get well. You've got a good reputation."

My reputation is made up of years of study, skill, training, experience, sleepless nights, tears, grey hairs, and fights with my wife about long hours away from home. And my reputation, really, is what I'm selling. You, the patient, are the customer. *You* are paying. And I like to think you pick me as your gastroenterologist because, on the recommendation of my peers, you know I can do the best job for you.

Meeting a new patient is fun for me. But sadly, few patients feel comfortable asking about my qualifications. Don't be ashamed. A good doctor should be proud of his training and experience, and eager to share it with you. If a doctor bristles at your questions, shrugs them off, or makes you feel silly for asking, smile politely and get out fast.

One day I had lunch with a friend, a portly gynecologist, who told me he had just learned a good lesson in humility from one of his new patients. Let's say her name was Anna Goldberg. He said, "What can I do for you, Anna?" She replied, "Sidney, I think I've got a vaginal infection." His eyebrows shot up. "You want to call me Sidney?'' he asked. ''Everybody else calls me Dr. Olan.'' She chuckled. ''Okay,'' she said, ''if you want to be formal, Dr. Olan, you may call me Mrs. Goldberg.''

My friend said he blushed, choked, and apologized. Since then, he's been ''Sidney'' to all his patients, and he asks their permission before he calls them by their first names.

You may not realize it at first, but a doctor who is friendly, relaxed, and respectful gives patients a lot more for their money. Not long ago one of my patients at Northside Hospital in Atlanta finally got up the nerve to tell me she was upset because, on morning rounds, I always *stood* by her bedside. She wanted me to sit down. So, I did. We had a pleasant chat, but I didn't stay any longer than usual. The next day she was beaming, thanking me for spending so much time with her.

This prompted my colleagues and me to conduct a little informal study. Several of us made a point of standing for two and a half minutes while we were in patients' rooms, and sitting for two and a half minutes, for our total and usual visiting time of five minutes. After a week we handed questionnaires to the patients, asking if they were satisfied with our visits. They all answered yes—because they thought we'd stayed *longer* than usual. The sitting down, face-to-face interaction did the trick.

But really listening to a patient's complaints is no trick. It takes some hard concentration. Sure, there are times I'd rather be out jogging, or having dinner with my wife, or even mowing the lawn. But I force myself to tune in to my patients as if each one is bringing me an exciting new medical jigsaw puzzle to solve. Making the diagnosis is such an intellectual challenge, as a matter of fact, that once in a while I get excited and forget I'm dealing with a feeling, caring, hurting person. That happened a couple of years ago. After weeks of tests and searching, I finally diagnosed a severe case of Whipple's disease. That's a rare malfunction of the GI tract, in which the patient cannot absorb nutrients; it's serious, and sometimes fatal. I went skipping down the hall, delighted with myself for being smart enough to pinpoint the disease, when all of a sudden I stopped short.

"My God!" I thought. "This is awful! I should be sad, not happy. This lady has a terrible disease."

I felt the bittersweet victory of a reluctant fox hunter: the chase was fun, but now it's over. I did a swell job . . . but the poor fox is dead.

I was ashamed of myself.

But I couldn't stay ashamed for long. Yes, I'm human too, but I won't do anybody any good if I don't maintain a high degree of self-confidence. Dr. Neil Kessel, physician and author, wrote an article in *The Lancet*, in May, 1979, called "Reassurance." In the article, he said that a doctor's confidence in himself in turn spurs hope and confidence in his patients, and helps them get well. I and other doctors must walk an emotional tightrope between tenderness and firmness, empathy and cool detachment. And through it all, I've got to make my patient feel that I'm 100 percent on his side: it's me and him against the illness . . . and we're going to win.

Once you feel you can win with your doctor because he or she has a personality that clicks well with you, half the battle is over. What's the other half? It's the doctor's brains and training, the sheer intellect needed to pull out every medical trick in the book to help you get well.

Gastroenterologists are specialists who have a lot of those "medical tricks" at their disposal. "Gastro" means stomach, "enter" means intestine, and "ology" is the study of it all. So, a gastroenterologist is a doctor who studies the stomach and intestines. All of us have three or four years of pre-med studies, leading to a bachelor of science degree. Then we go on to medical school (it takes about a B-plus college average to get in, and it's incredibly competitive) for four more years. At the end we've got an M.D., or medical doctor degree.

But it doesn't stop there. We've had our basic courses in anatomy, physiology, and the like, but we're far from being "real" doctors. We must first go through a one-year internship at a fine teaching hospital, to learn firsthand how disease affects people, and how it can be diagnosed and treated. Next, there's another two years of specializing in internal medicine.

Most of us are close to thirty by this time, but our training isn't over yet. We need two more years of a fellowship in gastroenterology, working in a medical school or hospital where gut diseases are seen, diagnosed, and treated every day. We also learn by going on rounds with senior physicians, attending conferences, and spending time in the laboratory.

During this extraspecialized training, we learn endoscopy. That's the use of special instruments, called "gastroscopes" or "colonoscopes," to see inside the stomach, intestines, and peritoneal cavity (the smooth lining of the abdomen). We also learn the delicate techniques of looking inside the colon—a procedure that takes a lot of skill, in order not to hurt the patient. Our training is extensive, and approved by the Federation of Digestive Disease Societies. It should be. We know that when you're on that hard examining table, with some young person in a white coat juggling steel tubes through your body, you want that person to be fast, artistic, totally in control, and very much able to make sense out of what he's seeing. You want an *expert*.

Doctors in training also work with older, more experienced men and women—experts—who supervise their education. My mentors were Dr. Eddy Palmer, who wrote *Functional Gastrointestinal Disease*, the classic in its field, and Dr. Howard Spiro of Yale University, who taught me how to listen to and care about patients. I think their intelligence and sensitivity got me started on the right track, and thinking of them gets me over a lot of tough spots in my day-to-day practice of medicine.

After about thirteen years of upper-level education and training, a gastroenterologist is finally ready to see patients of his own. But a good doctor, like any fine professional, never stops learning. I learn from every new patient, from hospital conferences, from meetings of local and national medical societies, from postgraduate courses, and from what seems like an endless number of medical journals. I belong to the American Gastroenterologic Association, the American Society for

Gastrointestinal Endoscopy, the American College of Gastroenterology, the American College of Physicians, the American Society of Internal Medicine, the Georgia Gastroenterological Association, the Georgia Society of Gastrointestinal Endoscopy, and several others. All this doesn't make me "superdoc," but it keeps me at my studies, and on my toes.

A patient who knows how active I am, not only in medical societies but in community affairs, asked me recently, "If you're so busy outside the office, how do you get time to see sick people?"

She made a good point. My answer is that it's another tightrope: I must, somehow, balance it all, and leave plenty of time for my wife, my three kids, and my personal friends. Now and then, somebody gets shortchanged. Yes, I sometimes keep patients waiting. Now and then they complain, and it does help me hustle. Maybe, while they were in my waiting room, I was on the telephone arranging for an evening out with my friends or talking about how to form an Israel bond committee. I've *got* to keep up those "outside" interests; I can't maintain my good humor and sympathy, patient after patient, without some breaks during the day for non-medical pursuits. Of course, in an emergency, my patients come first. My wife, with characteristic good humor, says that if she has aching guts, and a patient has aching guts, I rush to the patient first.

My patients know this. And you should know it, too, about your own doctor. Once you're satisfied that your gastroenterologist has the proper education and training, and that your personalities mesh well together, it's time *you* added a crucial ingredient: trust. Trust your doctor. Otherwise, chances for a happy, profitable relationship are slim.

The first thing your gastroenterologist will do is "interview" you in his office. He needs the answers to questions that help him figure out what's wrong with you—answers only you can supply. He must ask about everything from your mother's health (to determine a family pattern) to what you ate for dinner last night. Be totally honest with your answers, and don't be ashamed about anything. Nothing you say can shock the doctor; he's heard it all—and worse—many times before.

Next will come a physical exam. It should include everything from peering into your mouth to poking your abdomen, and perhaps examining your rectum with a thinly gloved finger. Relax. It's not great fun, but it's not terrible, either, and it's absolutely necessary.

Sometimes, a doctor makes his diagnosis after one visit. And sometimes blood tests, X-rays, and other diagnostic procedures are necessary before your doctor can say, "Now I know what's wrong." These tests are almost endless: they range from the familiar barium enema to "ultrasonography," a device that bounces sonar waves off your internal organs to detect possible abnormalities. There are also a variety of "little operations" that a doctor can perform to take out tiny bits of organ tissue, and test them in a lab. Finally, there is the ultimate but dangerous exploratory operation.

With all these diagnostic tools and techniques at his disposal, how does a doctor know when to quit? When does he figure out that you've had enough, and it's time to stop? When does he decide that "nothing is there," and you're having gut reactions?

It all goes back to what I've already said. If you picked your gastroenterologist carefully, his skill and experience tell him when "enough is enough." And, if you've done *your* part, such as answering all questions honestly and holding nothing back, your doctor will be able to arrive at a proper diagnosis within a reasonable amount of time. Again, trust him. He won't put you through expensive, uncomfortable, time-consuming diagnostic procedures for nothing. If you suspect or fear the doctor is being over-zealous in his search for an organic reason for your gut symptoms, sit down and talk it over with him. Your reluctance to go on with tests may be a way of saying, "Look, I know, somewhere deep down inside of me, that I have no disease, and I'm ready to explore the possibility of an emotional cause for my symptoms."

It's worthwhile to sit down and talk over anything on your mind that could possibly relate to your gut problems. If you've been abusing your body one way or another, tell your doctor about it right away. Don't blush, remain silent, and go through test after test just to have the doctor tell you what you suspected all along: that you drink too much coffee, or take too many enemas. Your doctor must know all the personal habits that might relate to your symptoms: what you eat, what you drink, what drugs, legal or otherwise, you use, and even if you chew on ice. Many patients are in great pain simply because they have what they think is the harmless habit of yanking an ice cube out of the freezer and munching on it. Sure, it has no calories—but it's murder on your guts. Drinking a lot of alcohol also turns your GI tract into a three-ring circus, but many patients are ashamed to tell me they're heavy drinkers, or alcoholics. I understand their shame, but it's foolish and dangerous to withhold that critical information from me. I'm not there to judge—only to help.

Many patients are also ashamed or reluctant to share their fears, whether it's fear of snakes, or elevators, or cancer. It can be a mild fear, or it can be a crippling phobia. Cancer phobia is very common, and the horrible, nagging fear that "I've got cancer" torments many patients. The fear itself can bring on cancerlike pain, especially if a relative or friend really has cancer, or has died from this disease. *Tell* your doctor about these fears. They're important in your diagnosis. Also tell about family fights or other domestic difficulties, sex problems, or job-related troubles. All this may or may not play a vital part in your symptoms, but you'll have a hard time knowing for sure unless you let the doctor in on your secrets.

You can see there's a lot of work involved in being a patient. It's up to you to choose the right doctor. It's up to you to cooperate in making the right diagnosis by sharing information with him. Of course, it's up to you to get through the tests with as much patience and good humor as you can muster. It's up to you to pay. And one more *very* important thing: it's up to you to follow your doctor's advice exactly. It's the only way to make sense out of it all; why go to such trouble and expense if you don't get the prescription filled, or alter your life habits as the doctor ordered?

What we doctors call the "compliance rate" of patients is enough to drive me up a wall. I invest a lot in every patient—just as the patient invests a lot in me—and I'm usually a mild-tempered, gentle fellow. I don't get flustered if you throw up in my waiting room, if you shout at my nurse, if you balk at having a needle jabbed in your arm, or if you call twenty times a day with questions. I am used to patients who are in a bad mood, who come late or who never show up for their appointments at all, who regard me with suspicion or dread, who have torn underwear, or who smell bad. Usually, none of that bothers me. But I will admit that I'm ready to tear out my hair when a patient puts me—and himself—through hell to find the source of gut trouble, and then refuses to follow my directions on how to get well!

Various medical studies show the "compliance rate" of patients is only about fifty percent. That means only about half my patients take their prescriptions *exactly* as I told them to, stop drinking, smoking, or whatever else I told them they needed to do, or went along responsibly and reliably with my medical advice. If you're that type of patient, there really isn't much I can do about it. Remember, I'm your doctor, not your mother. You may not like my advice, but if you don't follow it you've wasted your time and mine.

But if you do your job well as a patient, you can look forward to not being a patient for long. Your specific symptoms may never completely disappear, but you can learn to treat each one on your own, and erase the fear that often stabs at you when you're in pain.

The next chapter will help you learn how to manage some of the most common gut reactions so that you—not they—become the boss of your body.

5

Specific Symptoms

It often seems to gut reactors that they are at war with their own bodies. Their stomachs bloat and contract to devilish, unknown rhythms. Their guts churn as if they had a will of their own. Diarrhea, gas, vomiting, and pain come at the worst times: at a party, a business meeting, or in the middle of a meal. One patient sighed that, "I am two people—me and my guts. My guts are boss."

The art of healing the gut reactor is to reverse that situation and keep the guts under control. It's not easy. At first doctor and patient have to work together, testing a pill here, a hot bath there, a brisk walk, or a change in diet. None of the treatments is very complicated or remarkable, and little by little the doctor ought to back off and let the patient assume most of the responsibility for dealing with his symptoms.

The worst gut symptom is pain. In one way or another, it hits ninety percent of patients who have sensitive GI tracts. It can come in the esophagus, as a burning sensation in your throat; it can feel like a knife between your ribs when it affects your stomach; it can travel rapidly around the colon or lower abdomen like a spreading blaze; or it can throb through the rectum and around your back like the thump-thump-thump of a dreadful drum. Pain that is just an annoyance during the relaxed twilight hours can turn into a screaming tornado of discomfort in the stress of day. Some people can take a lot of pain; others become disoriented, tearful, or even hysterical when they feel the first twinge. It's subjective and highly individualized, and there often isn't much a doctor can do to help.

The pain of gut reactions is very real. Nobody "imagines" such agony. Researchers have put balloons into people's intestines and measured pain reactions on a recorder; they found the pain was caused mainly by abnormal intestinal contractions and distention when the sensitive patient gets upset. Some mysterious messages flash from the brain to the guts, and the guts respond by going into spasm: they contract. The worse the upset, the worse the contractions, and the worse the pain.

Why are some people controlled by their guts in this way? Other people don't take problems out on their guts at all: these people respond to emotional distress by shouting, or kicking the cat. Nobody really knows the answer. Dr. Don Powell, associate professor of medicine at the University of North Carolina, tried to pick out some differences between gut reactors and "normal" people in an article in *Gastroenterology* in 1973.

Dr. Powell said patients with the irritable bowel

syndrome registered a greater than normal "colonic basic electrical rhythm" on a monitoring machine. When the intestinal muscles contracted, the patient felt measurable pain. This shows the pain is *not* "all in your head" when you feel gut reactions. You might be said to have a "high colon pressure," just as some people have high blood pressure. Dr. Powell's research also showed gut reactors had increased colonic muscle pressure when they were exposed to various drugs, whereas other, nonsensitive people didn't react to the same drugs in the same way. The pressure also went up even when the spastic colon patient was resting—because his guts were active, even if he wasn't. And, of course, there were great changes in colonic pressure when the patients were subjected to emotional stress.

So the differences between gut reactors and people with "quiet" GI tracts, as measured by Dr. Powell, are there. But neither Dr. Powell nor anybody else can really explain *why*. The only honest way to put it right now is that for some unexplained reason, gut reactors have more "sensitive stomachs" than other people and when they get upset it turns into pain in the sensitive area.

Now you know as much as we doctors do. But that is not enough; you've got to know how to control the pain, and eventually stop it. Doctors can't do that for you.

Most doctors will prescribe some mild antispasmodics for their new gut reactor patients. Experiment with taking them the instant you feel the first twinges of gut pain. Maybe they will head off or reduce the contractions. In any event, you will feel more confident knowing that you have something in your system that might help. People who get pain very regularly, right after every meal for example, make a point of taking their antispasmodics on schedule. Perhaps they pop a pill just before each meal begins. The trouble with getting into a routine like this is you can become dependent on the drugs, both physically and psychologically, and you never get to the point of real mastery over your symptoms. You give the drugs credit for doing the job, when the credit should go to you. For that reason, patients who keep phoning a gastroenterologist with the same gut symptoms should get a gentle "no" from their doctors when they ask for more antispasmodic drugs. Eventually, you must, and probably will, learn to do without them.

You may want a really potent pain-killer like codeine to help you get through some ferocious attacks. But don't keep asking your doctor to refill this prescription, either. A heavy dose of pain-killer will further upset your already sensitive system, last much longer than your spasm, and probably give you a whopping headache. Some people just keep the pain-killer in their medicine cabinet; they say they feel better knowing it's there in case of an emergency, but they rarely use it.

You can train yourself away from pain. One patient I know of says aloud, "I'll give the pain thirty seconds." Then she counts to thirty, and it's gone. She plans to go down to twenty, and then ten, and five, and finally zero seconds for the pain. Another gut reactor, who used to double over with pain, forced himself to keep moving around "to show the pain that I could overcome the paralysis it imposed on me." At first, all he could do was crawl around the bathroom. Then he got up and took a few steps. He graduated to brisk walks through the house or down the office halls—wherever he happened to be when pain hit. Now, he jogs. A two-mile jog each day now keeps this middle-aged patient almost entirely pain-free. An older patient said she overcame gut pain by "talking to myself." When the pain comes, she says, "I say, 'This is coming because I am upset about something. I'll find out what I am upset about, and solve the problem. Pain, you are not solving anything for me, and you can't stay here. You are going to go away now.' " Her little "conversation," as she calls it, works almost all of the time.

The counting, jogging, and talking all serve the same basic function: they are a way of asserting mastery over your unruly guts. They turn attention away from the symptom—pain—to a more useful activity. They don't pretend the pain isn't there. They *control* it.

A good doctor rules out organic disease and gradually lets the patient assume control. That is why he should gradually withdraw drugs, respond more slowly to frantic phone calls, and gently discourage too many office visits. He has to get this message across: "Your body isn't sick, so I can't 'cure' it. You are the only one who can figure out the most effective pain control."

Of course, pain isn't the only major gut symptom. A lot of people have been to doctors' offices with complaints of what they call "gas." Patients say it feels like they are bloated, like they will burst, like little balloons are floating around their guts and blocking everything, and like they can't stop passing gas from the rectum or can't hold back frequent burping.

This, too, can be controlled. Passing gas in public isn't exactly considered dainty in the Western world, and we all stare angrily at children who do it on purpose and giggle over their accomplishment. When adults do it, we try to ignore the unpleasant sound or smell and pretend we didn't notice. But (to show this also is a function under your control) some cultures cultivate the art of passing gas. Belching was once considered a compliment in China, for example. Dr. Franz J. Inglefinger, an authority on gastroenterology, wrote in *Nutrition Today* in 1973 that "When Young-Low, Emperor of China (1403–1425), had finished his last bit of bird's nest soup, sulfurated egg and roast pork, and lay aside his chopsticks and dainty Ming bowl, he wanted to thank his host for the splendid feast. So he momentarily held his breath, squeezed shut his glottis, relaxed his upper esophageal sphincter, and with a series of diaphragmatic and thoracic muscular efforts, rapidly alternated his intrathoracic pressure between negative and positive values. The result was a mighty series of burps, delivered at a rate of about twenty a minute and only ceasing when his Imperial Highness had to stop to take a breath. The host was very pleased, for the Emperor eructated at that rate only when the gourmet in him was perfectly gratified."

When you burp or belch (pass gas orally), or suffer flatus or fart (pass gas rectally), and it gets out of control, you are having a gut reaction. That is bad enough, but the swollen, "stuffed up" feeling that comes with the symptoms is even worse.

The gas in your intestines is made up of nitrogen, oxygen, hydrogen, carbon dioxide, and methane. In small amounts, it floats through everyone's intestines, and is eventually expelled every now and then. Gut reactors do pass more gas than other people; it gets into their bodies when they gulp air out of anxiety, or when they are so "tied up" with constipation that colon bacteria get a chance to overmultiply.

A brisk walk is probably the best cure for gas. It stimulates the intestines to greater movement, pushes along the offending material, and propels it out of your system. Another way to control the gas problem is to watch and see if you are an anxious air-gulper. People who eat too fast, talk too rapidly or too much, or do a lot of "oh-ohing" are really gasping and taking in chunks of air. It's bound to make them feel bloated and uncomfortable. Keep your mouth shut, and breathe slowly through your nose. One patient who complained, "Everything I eat turns to gas" got relief by eliminating pork and beans from his diet. Keep a diary of what foods give you gas and experiment by eliminating these foods to see if that helps. Sometimes, the addition of certain bulk-forming foods such as bran will help eliminate flatus and burping.

The other most common gut symptoms—constipation and/or diarrhea, heartburn, nausea, weakness, and churning—usually go along with pain and gas. They may come and go, they may be almost constant, or they may disappear for weeks and then pop up at totally unexpected moments. *There is no specific or definitive treatment for any of these symptoms*. Common sense is your best weapon. If you get gas after eating onions, just eliminate onions from your diet. Don't ask your doctor *why* it happens. He doesn't know! If a hot bath can relax your churning guts, just sit in the tub. Don't insist this "cure" is too simple, and look for drugs instead. Use the bath. It's probably the best all-around symptom reliever we know. Take prescribed drugs only if you need them, and adjust the dosage to what you know your own body tolerates; get together with your doctor on this and make a joint decision. Always work toward self-treatment, self-reliance, and self-control of your symptoms.

Little by little, over a period of time, your object is to stop letting your guts rule your world. One forty-two-year-old housewife got terrible diarrhea whenever she dressed to leave the house. She traced the onset of her symptoms to the day she decided to look for a job. The diarrhea was a way of holding herself back—of staying in a boring but familiar routine. "I was terrified that I would get caught on the highway, in my car, and have to 'go,' " she said. "It got so bad that I'd scout for a street with a lot of gas stations so I could rush into the restroom if necessary. Finally, I decided it was ruining my life. I took a plastic bag with me in the car, thinking that if the worst thing happens, I'll just go in the bag. And I did. Nobody arrested me. Nobody even saw me! After that, the problem gradually diminished. After about seven or eight months, it went away."

Another gut reactor got severe pain whenever her boss congratulated her, or she won acclaim for her work. At first she simply stopped doing good work, but realized she was "giving in" to her guts. So she stayed on the job and gritted her teeth through the pain. She reported later, "It eased off and disappeared, but it took nearly two years. It was hard to go through that, but I feared the pain was going to keep me from ever gaining success if I didn't fight back."

The less you talk about, complain about, and worry about your guts, the better. It may be the same with other bodily malfunctions. Psychiatrist Melvin J. Stern, an associate professor at George Washington Medical Center in Washington, D.C., recently told an American Heart Association seminar that the best recoveries after heart attacks are made by "tough, self-reliant patients who don't worry about themselves." Male heart attack survivors did best when they went right back to work, engaged zestfully in sex, and didn't "become obsessed with physical symptoms." Females recovered from their heart attacks quicker if they, too, returned to work quickly. Housewives did best when their husbands didn't worry about them or do housework for them.

The same could be said for gut patients. When you constantly fret about what you eat, avoid potential stress to stave off gut pain, or keep away from parties because you may get nervous in a crowd and might get diarrhea, you are training yourself to "baby" your symptoms. Step out and plunge into activities. Don't let friends or family cater to your symptoms with special foods, or activities built around your "infirmity." Don't talk about your symptoms, tell your spouse when you've had a bad day, or cancel events when you feel weak. Don't lie down. Don't rush to the bathroom when you are nauseated. Take a sip of Coke instead, and try breathing slowly. One patient starts humming when he feels like he is going to vomit. He said it takes his mind off the nausea, and also has gained him a reputation among other workers as a "jolly fellow."

Now and then, your symptoms will get the better of you. But if you don't make a big deal out of it, neither will anybody else. People won't gasp in horror at a friend who has a bellyache or gets dizzy once in a while. That is viewed as normal. If it helps, check with your doctor each time this happens. In a recent double-blind study, gastro-enterologists throughout the country gave an anti-spasmodic to some patients who had gut troubles, and a placebo, or sugar pill, to others. They all got better! Why? It wasn't the real or fake pill that helped; it was the extra care lavished on them by their doctors. If you need that sort of attention from your doctor, and if it helps, by all means ask for it. But don't expect other people to give it to you. Spouses, children, friends, and coworkers will soon get tired of treating you like a baby every time you gasp in pain, belch, vomit, or get dizzy. Let your doctor, and *only* your doctor, reassure you about your symptoms. Then go on as quickly as possible to reassuring yourself, and relying on your own strength of character to overcome the symptoms.

You may have been born with a sensitive GI tract, but you learned how to use it to express anger, guilt, fear, or frustration. So, you can unlearn that, too, and direct your emotions to more useful and less painful ends. The change is important not only for you but for your family, because children will tend to pick up your gut reactions and start displaying the same symptoms. It's your responsibility—not your doctor's—to make sure you don't leave your kids a legacy of GI troubles. Also, a gut-reacting spouse, lover, parent, or grown offspring puts a strain on any relationship by becoming a dependent bore. Some gut reactors turn into terrible problem patients, too, thwarting the doctor's efforts to make them well and subconsciously prolonging their own pain. In the next chapter, I'll set out the warning signals that mean you're using your guts to brew up some trouble with your family or your doctor, or both. It's up to you to spot the signals in yourself, and work with your doctor on ways to stop them.

6

Gutsy Relationships

Some patients scare me. No matter what I do, their gut pain persists. I like most of these people, and my heart goes out to them; I keep muttering to myself, "I know there is nothing wrong. Why must they suffer so?"

They must suffer, it seems, because their aching guts serve an important function: they allow the gut reactor to control other people. A young lady who is frightened by sex can get horrible cramps when she crawls into bed with her lover—and he will quickly leave her alone. A wife who doesn't really want to cook dinner, but who feels obligated to do so, can double over with pain—and hubby will cook instead. A man who claims to want a new job but secretly fears the responsibility can stay in bed the morning of his interview, moaning and clutching his belly—and his wife won't nag. And all of these people can come to my office, ask endless questions, pepper me with pleas and complaints, and get my constant reassurance. Their guts are a one-way ticket to instant attention.

Gut reactors usually don't want things to work this way. The pain is real, and the reasons for it are quite subconscious. I'm not a psychiatrist, but my educated guess is that people with gut symptoms gradually learn, when they are children, that tummyaches can be a convenient way to avoid responsibility, escape fearful events, or punish parents. If the trick works, it's used again and again, until gut reactions become an ingrained personality pattern.

We can and usually do put up with some bellyaching from children. But as the bellyacher grows up, he or she becomes a terrible nuisance. Either nothing gets done because gut problems always interfere, or too much gets done and gut problems become the price of success. The whole family lives in dread of the patient's "attacks." Sadly, when the patient gets old enough to marry and has kids of his own, he almost "trains" them, also, to respond to life's stresses with gut reactions.

"It's a fairly widespread medical opinion that reacting in a somatic mode is passed on from parent to child," says Dr. Ralph Klopper, an Atlanta psychoanalyst. "When a mother or father has a stomachache or vomits when things go wrong, the child will probably do that too. It's a matter of models. The child identifies with his parent's behavior. He is learning to cope with life's problems from his best teachers: mom and dad."

Dr. Dan Caplan, a professor of pediatrics at Emory University's Medical School and a pediatric gastroenterologist at Georgia's Egleston

Hospital for Children, says, "There is no doubt that kids, even infants, quickly learn to take out their troubles through their tummies. I get a small patient with GI complaints and almost inevitably I find out that his parent or grandparent, or both, suffer these same symptoms.

"And I can tell right off the bat," Dr. Caplan adds, "that the children share their parents' neatness, their high expectations for themselves, their need to do everything and do it perfectly. Yesterday I saw a thirteen-year-old boy who has the most terrible abdominal spasms. He is a whiz in school, and he is also on the basketball team, and the football, track, and swim teams. He fits soccer in, too. Also, he is in the school band, and when he gets home he dashes to the Boy Scouts. Sundays he is in the church choir. That poor kid has to be constantly doing something with every free minute he has, and his parents are both the same way."

Dr. Caplan sighed. "This boy was trained to be a gut reactor. He and his parents must learn to relax."

Atlanta pediatrician Dr. Herb Alperin says it isn't easy to tell a child to relax. He talks to parents, too, and "I explain that we all have aches and pains in our bellies, but we can't let that stop us. We still have our jobs to do. A child's job is to go to school, but not to do *everything*. A child's job is also to make mistakes. That is how we learn. I tell kids with functional GI distress to ignore their tummies and just go on. The parent is always in the room listening, and he or she will often pop up and say, 'Oh, I have stomachaches too.' "

Dr. Charles Harrison of Georgia, who calls himself "just an old country internist," says that although he has never done a formal study on the problem, "I see a lot of patients in early adolescence who frequently channel their anxieties into their stomachs. I know their moms and dads gulp a lot of Maalox and Alka-Seltzer, and I think they are passing that pain on to their kids."

It's sad to hand your child the awful inheritance of gut pains. Although it helps a lot if you have a sympathetic doctor talk this over with the afflicted child, usually the only real help can come from you. If you stop exhibiting gut symptoms, chances are the child will stop, too. In stubborn cases, a child psychiatrist is needed, especially if the boy or girl is over eight years old and has forcefully adopted the gut-reacting habit. Dr. Pi-Nian Chang, a pediatric psychologist at the University of Minnesota, has even perfected a self-hypnosis technique for children with what he calls severe "stress-related" pain. The children first learn that pain will bring them no rewards. For example, a stomachache is no excuse for missing school. "We tell the school not to give medicine or send the child home," says Dr. Chang. Instead, the child can go to the nurse's office and use the relaxation techniques taught by Dr. Chang: concentrate on getting rid of the pain, relax your whole body, think of pleasant things, and tell the pain to go away. It takes from two weeks to four months for a child to get rid of pain this way, says Dr. Chang, and he must keep reminding parents and teachers that the children are not faking. "The pain is there," he says, "but the child can learn not to be incapacitated by it."

Gut patients who want to protect their children from a lifetime of pain and GI symptoms often force themselves to "hurry up and get well," so this doesn't happen. But it's more difficult to see how your guts can interfere with the lives of older family members. You usually don't transfer the pain to a husband or wife, but you do make them worry about you and give in to your demands. Eventually, they become frustrated and angry with the same old symptoms. One weary husband told me, "All I hear when I get home from work is a blow-by-blow account of what happened to my wife in the toilet that day. She is usually too sick to make dinner, and she might get sick if we go out to eat. It is getting so that when I see her come in the room, all I can think of is one big bellyache." One young wife told me she was thinking of asking her husband for a divorce so she could spare him nightly bouts with her weakness, pain, vomiting, and other gut reactions. He said no; he loved her too much to give up. She went to a psychiatrist instead, and got much better.

I'm proud of patients who fight their disability this way. To me, they are brave, determined, and smart; they want more fun out of life, they know they can get it, and they usually win. When I can help a patient like this—with a pill, with a pat on the hand, or with a reassuring chat—I feel good, too.

But there are a few patients who can make me frustrated and angry. I suspect their families could say the same thing, too. Some of these patients often make my heart sink when I hear their voices on the telephone; with others, I have the fantasy of running away when they walk into the waiting room.

In 1978, in an article in the *New England Jour-*

nal of Medicine, Dr. James E. Groves of the Massachusetts General Hospital described some similar feelings. The article was called "Taking Care of the Hateful Patient." Dr. Groves said that certain patients exhibit well-defined personality traits that arouse negative feelings in their doctors. In turn, their doctors struggle with the aversion, despair, or malice they feel toward the patient instead of concentrating on making him well. I often wonder if this isn't a clever subconscious trick on the patient's part to make sure some competent doctor doesn't root out and erase his pain.

One of the most frustrating patients I ever met came to me early in my career, when I wasn't experienced enough to know what to do. She was a twenty-year-old art student named Lana. She popped into my office one day with a big smile, a warm greeting, and a strange history of psychogenic vomiting. Lana's workup showed she was healthy, and when I told her the vomiting was probably a gut reaction she took the news well. She listened carefully, her pert, pretty face intent on mine, and asked intelligent questions in a calm, clear voice. We both agreed the vomiting would take some long-term care, and when Lana left I felt sure I could help her easily.

I was wrong. Two days after our first meeting, Lana sent me a note that said, "Thanks for your care and understanding." It made me glow . . . but it was a setup for the disaster that followed. Two more days went by, and Lana showed up again, this time with questions about diet and medication. She was still pleasant. Then came the phone calls, often three a day, with Lana's voice reaching a high pitch of hysteria and anger. She vomited.

She fainted. She didn't know *what* was the matter. Neither did I, but by that time I was asking my nurse to intercept Lana's calls. So, Lana telephoned me at home, again and again. After six weeks I was exhausted, and I jumped whenever the phone rang. Finally I called it quits, and angrily told Lana our relationship would have to be confined to brief office visits. I should not have gotten angry. She quickly found another doctor.

Dr. Groves calls this type of patient a "dependent clinger." Like Lana, the clinger starts out as a mild-mannered human being and gradually turns into a demanding, overbearing, inconsiderate monster. The clinger insists on explanations, reassurance, medication, and affection from the doctor at any time of the day or night. Is there a really sick patient in your office? The clinger doesn't care! She is on the telephone again, asking the same questions you answered a few hours ago. Are you home, finally, after a sixteen-hour day? Watch out! The clinger is calling, and she will chat endlessly. Are you sick yourself? The clinger won't notice. She is too busy telling you about her own problems.

It is easy to be overwhelmed by this kind of patient, and "turn off." I did with Lana. Now I know better. I gently but firmly put rigid controls on patients like this so our relationship isn't totally destroyed. With one woman, I even have a timer. I set it for ten minutes when I see her in the examining room, and I make my exit when the bell rings. That way, we both get some relief.

I was more experienced when I met Mark, who fits the mold of what Dr. Groves calls the "entitled demander." Mark was a top-notch attorney, forty-four years old, and the way he strode into my office marked him as an aggressive, "I-am-in-control-here" type of guy. Mark had nonspecific abdominal pain; two other doctors had tested him extensively and found no illness. I couldn't either. I told Mark he was probably having gut reactions.

Mark wouldn't accept my opinion, but he wouldn't leave me alone, either. He kept demanding more tests, a better evaluation, a more thorough exam. Once he stared at me and said, "It would be malpractice if I really had something bad, you know, and you missed it."

Mark made me feel guilty, afraid, and angry. He made me worry about my reputation; his threats were taking hold. One day something snapped in me. I told Mark that as his doctor I was sure of what I was doing, and that I was going to help him if he would get the chip off his shoulder and cooperate. Somehow, I recognized that Mark was playing the bully because he wanted to hide his deep dependency. We get along now, but he is still not one of my favorite patients.

One lady who seems destined to remain a patient forever is Melissa, a thirty-five-year-old college professor. She has had alternating diarrhea and constipation for twenty years, but is perfectly healthy. Melissa has also been on and off a psychiatrist's couch, but she never stays put long enough to really get at her emotional problems. She uses the same tactics on me: no matter what I do, Melissa makes sure it won't work. If I prescribe an antispasmodic, she forgets to take it. If I recommend a high-bulk diet, she substitutes a low-bulk diet. If I say, "Don't take anything," she plasters herself with drugs. After each episode, Melissa comes back in my office with a smile of victory and says smugly, "I didn't get better." If I make another suggestion, she will shrug and sigh, "We tried that before," or "It probably won't help." Now and then one of Melissa's symptoms will go away—and quickly be replaced by another.

Dr. Groves would define Melissa as the "manipulative help-rejector." Every doctor knows at least one patient like this. We call them "chronics," or "crocks." They frustrate us again and again because no matter what we do, the symptoms and the disease are always victorious.

The last type of "hateful patient" described by Dr. Groves is the "self-destructive denier." Jack, a fifty-four-year-old sports writer, is my most recent patient like this. He is a pleasant, chatty fellow, but he won't talk about what matters most: his heavy drinking. Jack suffers from terrible burning pains in his chest and throat, accompanied by almost constant discharges of bile from his GI tract up into his windpipe. I am sure his symptoms come from drinking, but Jack won't admit to touching a drop. I have to keep testing Jack for liver disease, because that is a real possibility in his case. Yes, I get frustrated when I see Jack pursuing his slow form of suicide, but I must remind myself that it is his life, not mine, and I am there as his doctor simply to offer whatever help I can.

These so-called "hateful patients" are hard to handle, both in a family and in a doctor-patient relationship. But they have taught me a lot. Now I can spot the patterns, identify the problems, and set limits on the patient's dependency. That way, I can usually maintain the doctor's appropriate role of sympathetic, supportive, and objective healer. It is no longer easy for patients to turn me into an angry, frustrated "daddy."

But gut patients aren't the only ones who can do this to their doctors. Any chronic illness sets the stage for a potential mixup in the doctor-patient relationship. It is so common, in fact, that many physicians need some sort of guidelines in dealing with patients like this. I use the guidelines set up by Dr. Douglas A. Drossman, of Chapel Hill, North Carolina, in his paper, "The Problem Patient," published in 1978 in the *Annals of Internal Medicine*.

First, I allow a patient to give me his history in his own way. Instead of a series of prearranged questions I simply ask, "What is the problem? Tell me about it." Both the patient and I learn a lot from the spontaneous outpouring that follows. Of course, I follow up with specific questions, such as "Do you feel pain after eating?" and "Does anyone else in your family have these symptoms?" Through it all, I maintain what Dr. Drossman calls the doctor's necessary "unbiased interest." I listen. I don't judge.

A thorough physical exam follows, and there is usually some sort of lab test, or workup, too. When the test results come back—and with the gut reactor, they are almost always normal—I avoid saying, "The problem is emotional." Instead, I say "It's functional," or "Emotion is one of the factors causing you to feel bad." Later on, if I keep being supportive, the patient will realize, on his own, the extent emotions play in his illness.

The next step is to set up regular office visits, to provide constant but not overbearing reassurance to the patient. The patient now has to accept the symptoms as a long-term problem, and so do I. My constant refrain is, "We can't 'cure' this right away, but let's work on it together."

Seeing the patient on a regular basis also gives me a chance to watch for new developments or symptoms: anything that might indicate the start of a new problem, or the end of an old one. If I have what Dr. James Groves calls "a hateful patient" on my hands, I am monitoring my own feelings during these visits, too, to make sure no hostility develops.

Most of the time, it doesn't. I have already said that gut reactors, for the most part, are bright, witty, and well-educated. I have fun being with them. Clearly, they are complicated human beings, and it is a great challenge for me, and for them, to work on the emotional and physical jigsaw puzzle they present. And I care about them. I care about what they eat, how they feel, and about what happens in their lives. I know emotions play a big part in any illness, and I firmly believe that my smile and steady hand give patients the boost they need to fight their disease.

Dr. W. Walter Menninger made that point in his article, " 'Caring' as Part of Health Care Quality," which appeared in 1975 in *The Journal of the American Medical Association*. That same *Journal* carried an article in 1927, "The Care of the Patient," by Dr. W. Peabody, which became a classic in its field. The article sums up how I feel about what I am doing when I put my heart and soul into relationships with my patients: "The good physician knows his patients through and through, and his knowledge is bought dearly. Time, sympathy, and understanding must be lavishly dispensed, but the reward is to be found in the personal bond which forms the greatest satisfaction of the practice of medicine. One of the essential qualities of the clinician is interest in humanity, for the secret of the care of the patient is in caring for the patient."

7

Diet and Drugs

Diet is a big part of caring for gut reactors—mainly because they ask so many questions about it. Sooner or later, I have to tell them that what they eat probably won't make much difference in their symptoms.

The primary functions of your guts, or intestinal tract, are to take in food, process it, absorb it, and discharge the wastes. So, it's understandable why physicians, scientists, dieticians, other health specialists and a lot of worried mothers have concentrated for centuries on food as a way of "curing" or easing the symptoms of gut reactions. Special diets for people with "sensitive stomachs" fill volume after volume in our medical libraries.

The trouble is very few of these diets make medical sense. Almost none of them have stood the test of time by working consistently to relieve gut symptoms. Now, many doctors like myself are telling patients with functional GI problems that as far as *those* problems are concerned, most foods won't help or hurt you much at all. What does help, or hurt, is the way you feel when you eat, and how you feel about the food you are eating. If you have been conditioned to think that lettuce ties your guts into knots, it probably will. But if you can coax yourself into eating sensible amounts of wholesome food in a relaxed atmosphere, you will find that lettuce, or almost anything else, presents no hurdles. I consider it a great victory when my patients learn to relax and enjoy all kinds of food, particularly if they come to me after years of being what I call "dietary cripples." A dietary cripple is a gut reactor who has been so restricted by fears or by the suggestions of well-meaning doctors that food becomes an enemy. The doctor suggests or prescribes diet after diet, without encouraging the patient to consider an "anything goes" alternative. So, you wind up thinking that many foods are bad for you, and the zest for life that comes with a hearty, adventuresome palate is soon lost. If I find a dietary cripple among my gut-reacting patients, I quickly tell him to start sampling all sorts of foods again, without worrying about the potential consequences.

It often takes a long time, and a lot of courage to sample different foods and discover your guts can handle just about anything. A lot of gut reactors put themselves on so-called "bland" diets, hoping that innocuous amounts of rice, white bread, boiled chicken, noodles, and green peas might "go down easily." They probably do, but a diet like this is boring and unnecessarily restrictive. If you have an ulcer or some other organic GI disease, such a diet may help. But if your symptoms are functional—if you are a gut reactor—pecking at food like a weak sparrow only reinforces your image of yourself as being sick. And that is just not true!

I tell my gut-reacting patients to eat whatever they enjoy in moderate amounts and sample new foods with gusto. Many of them are afraid to try anything new, and others say that time and time again, much-loved but "dangerous" foods will give them trouble. I suspect that the trouble comes, however, because wary patients expect it to come. You may have had pain right after eating broccoli, for example, but the broccoli probably didn't do it. That fight you had with a buddy during the meal is what caused the problem. Nevertheless, you associate broccoli with stomach pain, and the "eat—get sick—avoid the food" cycle begins. If this happens enough times, you can convince yourself that almost any food is off limits. That is a terrible way to live.

For example, many patients tell me that coffee gives them gas or stomach pain. But when they switch to decaffeinated drinks, the symptoms stay the same or even get worse. Pizza, beans, or beets give some patients trouble. One woman told me she gets sick just looking at hot dogs, because every time she eats one she suffers for hours. Very often a quick swig of some alcoholic drink will send a patient into gut spasms, and so will the overuse of any spices. Perhaps these foods, for these people, were once associated with some unpleasant experience. The only sensible thing to do, I tell my patients, is to pinpoint the foods that bother them, stay away from those foods, and enjoy everything else. This simple process works as long as you cross only a few foods off your list. If you must eliminate a lot of foods because you're afraid of them, you could wind up with vitamin deficiency as well as a dull palate and a restricted social life. Nibble at the "dangerous" food when you are alone and relaxed, and try to introduce it slowly back into your diet.

Again, don't try to figure out why certain foods upset you. There is no explanation for why hot dogs are one woman's Waterloo, and another woman's delight, even if both women are gut reactors. Food, especially for gut reactors, is a highly personalized, individualized, and subjective experience. You must determine your own food intake. Restrictive diets—bland, low fat, or otherwise— are the result only of years of opinion and tradition, and they remain unsupported by solid scientific evidence.

There is evidence, however, for the use of certain diets for people with specific *organic* GI diseases. Some gut reactors may have these "real" diseases, too, so it is wise to know what they are and why diet helps or hurts in these cases.

People with celiac disease, or nontropical sprue, must eliminate gluten and wheat from their diets. Celiac disease affects the absorbing powers of the small intestines, and a slice or two of wheat bread eaten by a patient with this disease can cause severe cramping and diarrhea. Once the wheat bread goes, the symptoms usually go too.

Lactase deficiency is another specific malady of the lining of the small intestines. In this case, the patient is missing the enzyme lactase, which breaks down milk sugar, or lactose. So when ice cream or milk is eaten, the patient gets cramps, diarrhea, and bloating. Again, get rid of the offending foods, and the symptoms disappear.

There are other forms of sugar intolerance which most often respond to low-sugar or low-starch diets. Problems with the pancreas, liver, or gallbladder may call for low-fat diets or some other dietary regulations. Hepatitis or Cirrhosis, which are serious liver diseases, usually are helped by a diet restricted in fat. And, in 1978, a team of researchers at the National Naval Center in Bethesda, Maryland, showed that coffee, orange juice, and tomato drinks cause trouble for patients with reflux esophagitis, or severe heartburn caused by organic problems. The researchers were Drs. Price, Smithson, and Castell, and they published their findings in the *Journal of Gastroenterology* ("Food Sensitivity and Reflux Esophagitis"). In these patients, said the researchers, the treatment was simple: Stay away from those three trouble-some items and if you must gulp coffee, for example, follow it with a drink of water. That will usually "flush away" the symptom.

You should never assume you have any of these organic problems unless your doctor can prove it by running tests and making an exact diagnosis. Otherwise, using a bland diet and restricting your food in any way in an attempt to quiet your troubled guts is, for the most part, just a waste of time. And, it isn't much fun.

"I never can enjoy food," a thirty-two-year-old patient told me several years ago. "Cooking, baking, making salads; it's awful, because I like to do these things but I never enjoy my own products. Also, I can't have a good time eating in a restaurant. I have to tell the waiter, 'Don't put sauce on that' or 'I have to have everything boiled, not fried.' I am always afraid if I eat one wrong thing I will get cramps right there in front of everybody.''

That patient is now thirty-nine years old. She eats everything, and enjoys it. It took us seven years of gentle experimenting with everything from spinach to Mexican Tacos before she was "liberated" from her association of food with gut pain. She can now eat heartily in restaurants, and because she is a professional woman with little time for home-cooked meals, this is important. Most of all, she says, the freedom from self-imposed food restrictions has made her realize that her guts are under *her* control. Yes, she has gained some weight. She was 92 pounds when I met her. She is now 98 pounds, so her "liberation" hasn't hurt her figure. Instead, she looks and feels much better.

I have one generally accepted piece of solid, tested, scientifically-sound diet advice for this woman and other gut reactors. It relates to the value of a high-fiber diet, and this advice probably extends to us all.

For the past decade, Drs. D. P. Burkett and Neal S. Painter of London have researched the relationship of a high-fiber diet to a variety of diseases, including functional GI tract spasms. The research probably started when the doctors noted that Africans, West Indians, and Asians who ate a high-fiber diet seemed immune to the irritable bowel syndrome. In addition, in a statistical analysis, people who suffered from monumental constipation, slow intestinal passage of food, and low bulk stools associated with their low-fiber diets were more prone to appendicitis, benign and malignant tumors of the large intestine, hemorrhoids, varicose veins, and other diseases. The doctors decided there was a real connection between low-fiber diets and some diseases, and said the diseases might be avoided by adding fiber to the diet.

So far, the evidence has convinced me. I eat bran cereal and bran muffins, and urge my patients to do the same. One study, in particular, was responsible for converting me and others in the medical community to the benefits of the high-fiber diet: a controlled, six-week trial with twenty-six patients with irritable bowel syndrome. It was done at the Bristol Royal Infirmary in England by Drs. A. P. Manning, K. W. Heaton, and R. F. Harvey, and published in the August, 1977, issue of *Lancet*, as "Wheat, Fiber, and Irritable Bowel Syndrome: A Controlled Trial." In this trial, patients experienced great improvement in their gut symptoms when they ate foods loaded with fiber, and doctors were able to see an objective change in the motor activity of the colon in these patients. No such improvement occurred on the low-fiber diet.

I notice a similar improvement in my own patients when they take my advice and switch from white to 100 percent whole wheat bread and other high-fiber foods. An excellent dietary addition is bran breakfast cereals such as All-Bran. You can munch on bran right out of the box, but it is dry, so I like it best sprinkled on foods or made into cereal. Unprocessed miller's bran, available in health food stores or larger chain groceries, is fine for baking and homemade cereal.

There is no standard dose of bran, but most people do well on three to six tablespoons per day. The idea is to add bulk to your stools, so that gut activity is gently aided by these natural foods. You must discover the right dose for you, but I recommend enough bran or wheat fiber so you can have at least one or two soft bowel movements each day. A few people do feel some distention or bloating, and pass a little more gas, when they first add bran to their diets. But these symptoms usually disappear. It may take two or three months for a gut reactor to get some symptomatic relief from a high-fiber diet, but it's worth the try. Stick to it; it's very important to give the fiber a chance to work. Fresh fruits and vegetables may also be valuable dietary additions. I tell patients to cut down on refined sugar intake, however. It isn't a healthful food in general, and refined sugar contains no fiber at all.

Adding fiber to your diet may help; it certainly can't hurt you. The addition of certain drugs, however, do hurt many patients, and I have learned to view drug therapy as a two-sided coin: drugs can benefit gut reactors when used with great care, but they can destroy your guts, and maybe your life, if abused.

Like diet therapy, drug therapy is largely unproven. Some doctors and patients swear that certain drugs quiet their spastic GI tracts, and maybe they are right. But no solid, scientific evidence exists to show that any drug works consistently to help gut reactors. In 1975, researcher K. J. Ivey reviewed 400 papers on 18 different antispasmodic drugs, and couldn't find a single well-controlled study to prove that any drugs, given orally, eased gut spasms. The review was published in *Gastro-enterology* in 1975, and was called "Are Anti-cholinergics of Use in the Irritable Colon Syndrome?" As far as I'm concerned, the answer is no.

Still, I do prescribe these drugs now and then. Why? Because in *some* patients they seem to help *some* of the time. An anticholinergic, or anti-spasmodic, is simply a drug that blocks the nerves which probably cause colon spasm. If that seems to be the predominant problem in a gut-reacting patient, I will try an antispasmodic. Many of these drugs are premixed with mild sedatives or tranquilizers and this may be the reason why they work. But I prefer to give antispasmodics and tranquilizers separately, so I can control the dosage for each individual patient. If you accept an antispasmodic drug, ask if it is mixed with a tranquilizer. I think it is better to take them separately, if you take them at all, because chronic functional discomfort can quickly hook you on tranquilizers.

Remember that neither tranquilizers nor anti-spasmodics can "cure" your gut symptoms; they can only alleviate distress now and then. You already know the real reason for your symptoms is related to stress. For that reason, your doctor may try a mood-changing drug on the theory that if you can get relief from the depression or the anxiety caused by stress, you might also get relief from gut symptoms.

The most common mood-changers are the "so called" tranquilizers, with brand names such as Valium®, Librium®, Ativan®, Miltown®, and others. In most patients, they have a calming effect, and temporarily give a better chance at coping with life's strains. If you are in a mood where a broken vase seems like a major tragedy and you scream at the children for hours because of it and then wind up vomiting, the tranquilizer may help you put things back in perspective, at least for a while. If you are too depressed to scream, and come to me because of weakness, listlessness, and a general "what-does-anything-matter" attitude along with gut pain, I may prescribe an antidepressant. These drugs, known by the brand names of Elavil®, Tofranil®, Vivactil®, Sinequan®, and others are "mood-elevators," and may pep you up enough to fight your symptoms in a constructive way. Like any drug, they should be used judiciously, temporarily, and with a view toward helping you get over a particularly bad bout with gut symptoms so you can function in everyday life. Again, none of the drugs are for permanent use, and none of them provide a cure.

On a long-term basis, I'd rather stay away from mood-changers and prescribe specific drugs for each specific gut problem. Paregoric, Lomotil®, and Imodium® may provide temporary relief of diarrhea, but shouldn't be used if you have associated constipation, too. Recently, some medical researchers have suggested that irritable colon may be related to the abnormal release of a complicated substance, prostaglandin, in the intestinal wall. The researchers said a prostaglandin inhibitor might be helpful in treating gut reactors, and the best drug for this purpose is common aspirin. More specifically, a physician who had lactose intolerance reported taking some aspirin before he ate ice cream, and he didn't suffer his usual cramps as a result. So, aspirin or some of the newer and more complicated nonsteroid, anti-inflammatory drugs such as Naprosyn®, Motrin®, Indocin®, and others might be helpful for people who are having cramps, but who don't have ulcers, too.

For patients with duodenal, peptic, and gastric ulcer disease there is a ray of hope for relief in the form of a new drug developed in London by Smith, Kline, and French Laboratories. The drug, cimetidine, has the brand name of Tagamet. The drug is a potent weapon against the body's production of gastric acid and may be a major step toward an ulcer cure. It won't help people who only have gut reactions or functional and not organic pain, but it will help people who have both ulcers *and* gut reactions.

Over-the-counter laxatives almost never help, and they can really hurt people with sensitive GI tracts. In my opinion, they should be available by prescription only. Presently, nonprescription laxatives come in four categories: lubricants, bulk, saline, or irritants. Lubricants, usually mineral oils, can be used with discretion without much danger, but only in the proper, hospital-trained hands. Bulk laxatives, like Metamucil®, Effersyllium®, and Konsyl® (all trade names), might be helpful when closely supervised by a physician. The generic, or non-brand names for these bulk laxatives is *psyllium hyrophilic muculloid*.

Stool softeners, like bulk laxatives, are also reasonably safe. Trade names for some stool softeners are Colace®, Senekot®, and Dialose®. Their generic name is *dioctyl sodium sulfosuccinate*.

Study the names, and remember them. You need

this information if you're going to take care of yourself and become a wise medical consumer. Saline cathartics like magnesium sulfate are safe if used according to a doctor's directions. The most dangerous laxatives are the irritants: cascara, castor oil, or drugs containing phenolphthalein. These laxatives irritate the intestinal tract in an attempt to speed up the process of elimination. But in the attempt, the irritants cause gut spasm, cramping, and pain—just the symptoms you want to avoid! There are probably fifty or more of these irritant-containing laxatives on the market that you can buy without a prescription, and I put them in the category of "abused drugs." If you can, stay away from nonprescription laxative drugs. If and when you do select one, be sure to read the label and if you see an irritant like cascara listed, choose something else!

Antacids, antinausea drugs, or any item advertised as an aid to digestion should also be viewed as marginally effective and a possible danger, and used only if your doctor says okay. Even if he or she gives a thumbs-up sign to these preparations, use them with care and only on a now-and-then basis. Remember, your objective in the use of any nonnaturally-occurring substance is to obtain temporary relief, and not to become dependent on it. For example, some well-meaning doctors will prescribe pain-killers such as codeine to help you over a particularly rough time in your life, but people with chronic pain (gut reactors) are prime candidates for drug addiction. So, use drugs when necessary, but be careful.

Be especially careful to avoid some so-called nondrug related "aids to digestion" which are still on the market today, but which may damage even the most sturdy GI tract. Keep away from enemas; they should be used only in a hospital as part of a preparation for diagnostic procedures. I am still horrified when I run across an advertisement for "colon therapy" which I can only guess is the forceful introduction of liquids into the rectum for the purpose of cleaning out the colon. Recently such an ad in a little "health" magazine suggested that such therapy was a cure for constipation, fatigue, headaches, indigestion, and even overweight. Nonsense! The only thing such therapy might do is rupture your colon. There are still spas in Europe and in the United States which advertise "high colonic irrigations," and I can't imagine why anyone would want to subject their bodies to such worthless indignity.

I also tell my patients to avoid food additives, vitamins, wax preparations, or other store-bought potions. If you think you need something special to help you control your guts or to help your body in some other way, ask your doctor for a recommendation or prescription. Your doctor has taken the oath of Hippocrates, the father of medicine, who declared in 400 B.C. that physicians must "abstain from all intentional wrongdoing and harm, especially from abusing the bodies of man or woman . . ." Sellers of over-the-counter diets and drugs aren't bound by that oath. They may not wish to harm you, but it is possible their need to sell products might interfere with good judgment.

The very careful use of diet and drugs to treat gut reactors all boils down to this: we have no easy answers. It would be wonderful if some miracle food or pill could erase your pain or churning, but miracles are in short supply. So the best course of action, I think, is to try different foods, eat sensibly, and go easy on alcohol, coffee, fatty meats, candy, and other items everybody knows aren't particularly good for you. Try different drugs, too, as long as you are carefully supervised by your physician, and you don't let yourself get addicted to any of them. Stay away from food and "health" fads that promise quick relief but will probably only deliver more trouble.

And remember that diet and drugs are only one part of your overall life-style. They can't and won't do the trick alone. We will explore your style of life in the next chapter, with particular attention to charting a course for gut reactors that can offer as much enjoyment as possible in everyday living. Once you adopt a reasonable life-style, I hope you will learn to eat just about any food, and throw away every pill in your pocket.

8

Life-style

The term "life-style" is all-embracing. It covers the way you manage all daily duties and pleasures, from brushing your teeth in the morning to producing your company's annual report that afternoon, and then deciding what movie you'll see after work. Life-style also encompasses how you *feel* about all the large or small activities you do routinely, and how you handle unusual or unexpected events in your life such as a vacation trip, the birth of a child, or the death of your best friend. Life-style is the whole fabric of your life, and if you're a gut reactor it probably needs careful examination and some gradual but forceful changes.

Two critical components make up the sum of your life-style. The first component is external factors, or "outside" events such as accidents, death, or other people's activities over which you have no control. The second component is internal or "inside" factors, which is your ability to understand and constructively cope with the outside events. Everything that happens to you in life, everything making up your life-style, is a delicate combination and balance between these two factors. To imagine the interplay between "outside" and "inside" factors, picture yourself standing straight up, with your arms stretched out on either side, and your hands palm up. Now picture three small stones in each cupped hand. One hand holds the outside factors; the other, the inside factors. As long as they remain balanced, you're okay. Like a scale, you won't topple to either side if the weights are equal on both sides. But suppose something happens to unbalance the scale? Suppose you suddenly lose your job? A giant stone is plopped into the hand holding the outside factors, and unless you can quickly equalize the weight by adding a heavy dose of understanding on the other side, you're bound to get off balance.

Life is a constant struggle to keep that human scale reasonably balanced. Nobody I know achieves perfect balance all the time, but most successful and happy people manage not to lean too far in either direction. And, if they do, they can correct the imbalance pretty fast. Gut reactors seem to have a harder time keeping that balance. When an unexpected event or "weight" takes them by surprise, they might react not with an equal measure of constructive action to offset the strain, but with psychosomatic symptoms which further upset their scale of life and make it even more difficult to stand upright again.

The constant pulling, changing, shifting interplay between outside and inside factors—the constant jangling of the human scale—is something I like to call *dynamic tension*. The term is generally well-known among psychologists and other medical workers. Infants and children spend much of their lives subconsciously searching for a comfortable balance of dynamic tension. In adolescence and early adulthood, the search sometimes becomes desperate, which may be one reason why young people seem to suffer most from gut reactions. By the time you hit middle age, you've either found the level of dynamic tension best suited to you, or you constantly manifest the imbalance with some sort of signal for help. The signal could be alcoholism, headaches, gross obesity, overt aggression, a sulky, withdrawn personality, or gut reactions. You can use one of these signals or a combination of several of them, and once you've decided on a signal it rarely appears for the first time after middle age. For example, gut reactions hardly ever show up as a new complaint in a patient over the age of fifty.

You can change both your levels of dynamic tension and your unpleasant stress signal. How? By changing the way you live.

Any change begins with the belief that the change is both necessary and worthwhile. One of my biggest jobs as a doctor is convincing people that the seeming "little things" I tell them to do will really make them feel better. The advice to take a brisk walk every day is a good example. Sophisticated patients who come to me bloated and cramping, and who've spent enormous amounts of time and money on office exams and lab tests, will frown with disbelief when my "prescription" turns out to be a half-hour walk around the block. It seems too simple! Instead of accepting my suggestion for this change in life-style, they might leave my office grumbling with anger. Sometimes it takes me quite a while to explain how a walk might be the extra good "weight" they need to balance the "inside factors" side of their personal scale. They might not realize the walk could gradually become a coping mechanism, to replace gut malfunctions. If the person listening to me is trusting, cooperative, patient, and willing to try anything reasonable in his quest for relief, he'll change his life-style to include a daily walk. If he's skeptical, impatient, and insists on instant, dramatic results, there may not be much I can do to help.

Some patients refuse to change their lives in any way, large or small, because they *need* their symptoms. Dr. Lawrence S. Miller, medical director for the Rehabilitation Institute of Glendale Adventist Medical Center in Glendale, California, says that some people cling to chronic pain for subtle psychological reasons such as avoiding unpleasant jobs, getting attention from a spouse, or as a reason for neglecting their children.

"It should be clearly understood that these people are not malingerers," Dr. Miller told a reporter. "It is easy for a physician to spot a malingerer or a hysteric. The need to keep one's pain is far deeper than that. It may be a wife who has an atrocious marriage. She is ignored and belittled by her husband. When she has pain, he is sorry. He takes her out to dinner. She is important because she suffers."

Dr. Miller's point is that while the suffering of bodily pain may not be coming from any organic cause, it is quite real: the patient feels it as keenly as if he had been sliced with a knife. In gut reactors, the pain may take a variety of forms. Nobody knows why one patient is crippled with cramps, while another might suffer nausea and belching. It's also a mystery why some patients manifest just gastrointestinal symptoms, while others get hit with chest pain or headaches, too. I've noticed, in my own patients, a high correlation between gut problems and headaches. In many people, they apparently go together.

No matter how many symptoms are present, and no matter how bad they are, most people who are determined to get rid of them usually accomplish that goal. Dr. Miller says people with a good "outlook on life" refuse to give in to pain.

"We see it every day," Dr. Miller declares. "We see those with much to gain manage their pain; those without cannot do so. Everyone knows successful people who have had terrible debilitating illnesses and injuries and they move ahead with their careers. It is their conditioning to life which gives them the will."

Your "conditioning to life," or programming, as some psychologists call it, starts very early. I believe you begin feeling both the strains and the pleasures of life while still in the womb. The regular heartbeat, gentle movements, and rich nutrition of a relaxed mother must provide a very different intrauterine environment as compared to the palpitations, churning, and possible infusions of drugs and cigarette smoke imposed upon a fetus by a mother who is nervous or unhappy. Later, the touching, smiling and feeding you get as an infant give you your first overall ideas of what to expect from life. You subconsciously know if it will be calm, joyful, and filled with fun, or inconsistent, troublesome, and laden with one sad event after another. By the time you're four or five, I believe, the conditioning or programming probably hits its peak, and you've developed some rudimentary coping mechanisms. For some people, the lucky ones who've had pleasant programming, that coping mechanism could be a grin and a cheery, "I'll keep trying." For others, it could be gut reactions.

Usually, the conditioning isn't one-sided. Most of us have childhoods filled both with hugs *and* spankings. Frequently, a gut reactor will also have that cheery grin and determined attitude. Those are most often the people who beat their symptoms!

Conditioning never stops. We're programmed by parents when we're very young, but as we grow we are influenced by teachers, clergypeople, friends, doctors and lawyers, movie stars, and even by books, magazines, newspapers, radio, and television. The mixture of all these influences has a profound effect on how we seek to balance our dynamic tension, and a doctor who listens carefully to how a patient looks at his world can usually pick up clues as to where the imbalance might be. One of my favorite patients, a heavy-set black man in his early thirties, told me he was puzzled because his "stomach acted up" at the most unexpected moments. He had pain, he said, when he was relaxing at a baseball game, when he munched popcorn with his kids, or even when he walked his dog. "When you'd think I'd get sick, like when I'm under heavy pressures on my job or when I have a fight with my wife, I do okay with my stomach," he said. "But just when it seems I'd be calm and relaxed and having fun, I'm running to the bathroom or nearly crying with pain."

It took several long discussions before both my patient and I realized that he had been programmed by hard-driving parents to constantly clutch at power, wealth, and a leg up the social ladder. Relaxing made him feel guilty. His well-meaning parents, who worked hard to overcome racial prejudices by educating their children and pushing them into upper-class lives, probably never dreamed they had not equipped their son to understand his success drives, or temper them with an equal drive toward pleasure. When he finally decided this imbalance was causing more pain than he wished to tolerate, my patient gradually cut down his working hours and gave in to a long-denied simple pleasure: he started a rose garden. For him, this was a major change in life-style. As the roses bloomed, so did his ability to engage in noncompetitive, relaxing activities without paying the price of a gut reaction.

In the past, doctors assumed blacks rarely suffered from stress-induced discomforts like gut reactions, because few blacks were treated for the symptoms. But now I think we're beginning to realize being black has often meant being poor, and poor people don't always get the same careful medical attention as do the rich. So, the stress-related problems of the poor were, and still are, often ignored.

In my own practice, I see many upwardly-mobile, hard-driving black men and women determined to shatter the stereotypes and plunge into middle and upper-class lives. They suffer the same gut problems as overanxious whites and their relief often comes in the same way: with a change in life-style.

One priceless treasure possessed by my rose-gardening patient—and by other patients who successfully beat their gut symptoms—is his generally happy outlook on life. He has his problems, as we all do, but his basic attitude is that life is worthwhile and worth living to the fullest. On December 16, 1979, *The Wall Street Journal* reported Dr. George E. Valliant of the Harvard-affiliated Cambridge Hospital in Massachusetts had done a study on 188 Harvard men, and found the men who were happy led healthier, longer lives than the men who were unhappy. Men who showed successful "adult adjustment" and enjoyed their marriages and jobs stayed fit and free of significant disease in middle age. But men who were divorced, bored or frustrated with their jobs, or unable to enjoy recreation tended to suffer from cancer, heart disease, high blood pressure, and other illnesses by the time they were fifty-three years old. Dr. Valliant's analysis seems to give some solid scientific backing to what we all may already have suspected: that the happier you are, the longer and better you will live.

There are loopholes in the study, of course. For one thing, Harvard folks aren't representative of the general American population. But my most serious quarrel with this and similar medical research projects is that they tend to be done on men. Most of my gut-reacting patients—about sixty-five or seventy percent—are women. In talks with other physicians, I find they, too, treat a higher percentage of gut reactors who are female.

To my knowledge, there are no specific studies that pinpoint irritable bowel syndrome as mostly a woman's disease, but researchers do mention that women more commonly display gut reaction symptoms than do men. On November 4, 1972, *The Lancet* reported that "Unexplained abdominal pain is the tenth commonest cause of hospital admission in men and sixth commonest in women." And in "The Irritable Colon Syndrome," published in 1962 in *The Quarterly Journal of Medicine*, two doctors describe gut reactors as people who are "unable to take life calmly," and point out that most of these people happen to be female. These women are not poor, worried about cancer, or losers in the game of life, say the doctors. And, they're in good physical shape. They're just nervous almost all of the time. So, according to the doctors, the women use their stomach distress "to represent a particular mode of responses to a difficult life situation."

Women, perhaps, have traditionally had less of an opportunity than men to complain about or extract themselves from a "difficult life situation." In the past decade life has improved immeasurably for women in the United States, thanks mostly to the women's liberation movement. But females are still, by and large, conditioned or programmed to passively accept and swallow life's injustices. They may pout, nag, gripe, or get "bitchy" (all the traditionally acceptable, if nasty, hallmarks of the unhappy female) but many males are still terrified of a woman who calmly sizes up an unpleasant situation, chooses a rational and constructive alternative, and then follows through on her decision. I suspect that to one extent or another we all still consciously or subconsciously teach our little girls that they're more "feminine" if they accept a boring job, a wandering spouse, or an abusive acquaintance than if they firmly compete for a promotion, confront the spouse, or tell the annoying companion to "buzz off." So they bottle up the rage, confusion, anxiety, and bitterness, and let it out in another socially acceptable way: they get a stomachache.

Changing this deeply ingrained pattern, which I see most often in females, takes a lot of insight and effort from both doctor and patient. Courses in assertiveness training, group therapy with a reputable counselor, or any other insight-gaining experience is often helpful. Not all gut-reacting women are passive, under-the-thumb-of-hubby types. Many of them are highly successful business people who exude radiant good sense and a high degree of self-dependence.

Passive women, however, are easier to explain as gut reactors. Most often they're cheery little housewives on the outside and boiling infernos of anger inside. They're often married to hard-driving, domineering men who derive great security from keeping a tight lid on "the little woman," although the men are rarely aware of their destructive attitudes. They say they love their wives, and want to "protect" them—except the wife is hungry for a chance to escape the suffocation of such blind protection. At the same time, these passive women rarely get along well *without* a paternalistic male. They both resent and depend upon their overbearing "daddies," and if they would agree to psychiatric treatment, it would probably take some time before they learned the joys of self-reliance. Often, these women don't work well with me, because I'm not a "daddy-type" doctor. I don't shield them from bad news, call them cute names, or expect their husbands to pay the bill. After a few visits, these women often drift away to a more paternalistic doctor.

Women who are assertive, competent, successful, and sure of themselves are easier patients for me. Their gut symptoms may be a long-standing habit—a holdover from a repressive childhood they've now overcome—or a coping mechanism representing their last symbolic submission to a male-dominated society. These women usually aren't afraid to give up their symptoms, and they're eager to try almost anything to find relief. One patient discovered her vomiting went away after she told her husband she really didn't want to cook dinner after working all day. He balked at sharing kitchen duty, but she insisted, and they finally compromised by hiring a cook. Another patient, who is an attractive executive in her late forties, found relief from intense gas pains after meals when she sweetly but firmly told her boss that she, not he, would decide when she took her lunch break. And a young accountant erased her own crippling gut pain by making a much bigger change in life-style. She quit her dead-end job and renovated a room in her home as a private office, so she could begin a career as a consultant. "The pain went away for good, I think, when I put a lock on the door of that office and got up the courage to tell my husband and children that it was all *mine*," she reported. "Until then, I'd really felt guilty about using up a whole room in the house just for me."

Whether it means changing your eating habits, your place of work, or the way you relate to other people, *some* change in life-style usually is necessary to cope with gut reactions. The change may bring full or partial relief, but it usually should be done gradually, firmly, and with an eye toward relieving symptoms, not conquering worlds or wreaking vengeance on repressive friends or relatives. Life-style changes most often require the help of a physician, and if I can't handle the job alone with my patient, I will refer that patient to a competent psychiatrist or psychoanalyst. Somatic manifestations of deep-seated depressive disorders often need long-term analysis and treatment, and I'd be most likely to recommend a psychoanalyst, who is an M.D. with special training in psychiatry and who has undergone the analytic process. Patients who benefit most from analysis are usually bright, well-educated, capable of and interested in self-analysis, mature enough to commit themselves to long-term treatment, and determined to live a fuller life. Analysis can cost as much as $100 per hour, but many clinics and young practitioners are considerably cheaper. Fees also vary from state to state.

Perhaps one of the greatest benefits of analysis or intensive psychiatric care is the "live and let live" attitude it fosters in patients. Gut reactors, especially, tend to be perfection-oriented people who like to control not only themselves, but almost everyone around them. When I describe a gut reactor in my medical files, I often find myself using the words "domineering," "manipulative," "compulsive," or even "bossy." Making sure the world functions correctly is an overwhelming responsibility, yet gut reactors often assign that job to themselves, and take it all very seriously. They want to "reform" everyone, eliminate social problems, and erase everything from vandalism to global war. One forty-three-year-old fashion consultant said she couldn't be happy until everyone in her city "dressed right." That meant, of course, everyone must dress *her way*—and it also meant since this would never happen, she was really saying she could never be happy. But she kept trying to impose her fashion ideals on everyone she knew, and also manifested the trait of trying to dictate nearly every movement made by her husband and children. At the same time, the patient doubled over with cramps at almost every social function she attended, because she felt it was her fault if people were poorly dressed.

The fashion consultant finally left her gut reactions behind after three years of psychoanalysis. She also told me she abandoned the need to watch her husband's diet, set out her daughter's clothes in the morning, or supervise the way her son cleaned his room. "How relaxing it is," she chuckled, "to let them live their own lives. Now the only person I have to worry about is me, and it feels great!"

An analyst is usually necessary to achieve a major personality change like this. But with or without an analyst, a commonsense life-style is easy to describe. Ideally, it revolves around a healthy sense of self-respect, a satisfying network of family relationships, a creative and rewarding job or career, proper nutrition based on a low-fat, high-bulk diet, prudent or no use of drugs and alcohol, no cigarette smoking, a proper balance of work with play or hobbies, and at least one purely physical outlet such as jogging.

We humans are physical creatures; we are, after all, animals. And animals were never meant to sit still all day, or to allow any event to make hearts pound and guts churn without getting up and making some physical movement. Wild animals know what to do about stress: they fight, or run. But what do we humans do? Too often we sit still, bite our fingernails, and get a bellyache.

I prefer running. Both partners in this book, David the physician and Maxine the journalist, are runners. We cover about three miles in 25 minutes at a time, and we do it three times a week. We're running toward some exciting goals: fitness, relaxation, a sense of drama and achievement, communion with nature, and the potent relief from gut problems that running affords for us. Running is inexpensive (all it takes is a good pair of athletic shoes), can be done anywhere and at any time, and requires little style, training, or talent. Running is a particularly good sport for relieving tension because it's so informal. There is also a great sense of comradery among runners if you choose to run with others. Even if you start off alone, you get a wave of the hand and a nod of recognition from other runners you pass on the street. You can join them if you wish, then break away again. Running doesn't require explanations, appointments, or excuses. You don't have to cope with selecting gear or equipment, or showing up on time for a reserved court or field.

Running, jogging, or brisk walking helps almost every gut reactor willing to incorporate this simple physical activity into his life-style. The rhythmic movement may provide the perfect "medicine" to calm writhing guts by providing relaxation, and also by moving along any trapped gas present in the colon and abdomen. Dr. George Sheehan, in his *Running and Being—The Total Experience*, even declares that running can help a determined person accept and overcome some organic disabilities. "There is hardly anything right going on in my abdomen," he says. "How could it with a hiatus hernia, a duodenal ulcer, an absent gallbladder, diverticulosis, and two sizable inguinal herneas?" Yet this abdomen doesn't stop Dr. Sheehan from enjoying life, at least partly through the experience of running. He adds, "The runner–doctor knows that health has nothing to do with disease. Health has to do with functioning and wholesomeness and reaching your level of excellence. My health has to do with my life-style . . ."

If running isn't your idea of a great life-style, try swimming or simple gymnastics. For some, tennis or golf provide the answer. Generally, the best prescription is what works for you, but I urge my gut-reacting patients to try a sport that doesn't require being competitive, making appointments with people, or engaging in elaborate preparations.

Two years ago a slender, twenty-nine-year-old patient who was an avid skier told me sadly that he had to abandon his sport because "getting prepared with all the gear is such a hassle." He described the anxiety that crept over him as he pulled on layer after layer of skin-tight clothing, buckled his cumbersome boots, adjusted his skis, and inched along in the lift line. "By the time I was scooped up in the lift, man, I'd be a nervous wreck," he said. "I could just feel the churning inside. I'd sit there with my skis dangling and just pray that I didn't get diarrhea. Once I got off the lift and started down the slopes it was wonderful. But, oh, the preparation for it all almost wiped me out!"

I told this young man to pack away his ski gear for a year or two, and substitute jogging. He did. And not long ago he told me, during his annual physical exam, that he was ready to ski again. "I think I can take it in a more relaxed way now," he grinned. "I feel more confident about controlling my guts because I never got diarrhea when I was running. And, Lord knows, when I run I'm miles away from the nearest bathroom, just like when I'm skiing."

Such recognition and confidence is an important change in life-style for my skiing friend. He thanked me for the advice about running, and I thanked him for teaching me it's possible to suspend an activity which you enjoy but causes you stress until you learn how to cope with that stress. Then, like the skier, you can renew the activity. Still, I know that of all the sports and activities I recommend, running is the one that works best for gut reactors. How do I know? The runners are usually the ones who don't need to come back so often to see me at the office.

9

Times of Trouble

A reasonably tranquil, well-balanced life-style seems to be the key to managing gut reactions, and I am convinced this can be achieved if you are determined and patient enough. But what happens when trouble comes your way and temporarily or permanently changes that life-style? Nobody can sail smoothly through life without a storm swirling around them now and then. These storms, in the form of troublesome life-altering situations beyond your control, often bring on gut reactions.

All major life-cycle events can be times of trouble: career choice or change, marriage, pregnancy, birth, divorce, illness, or death. Sometimes these events are joyful; at other times they seem like disaster. They can be happy or sad, but when an event changes your life in any significant way, that can be troublesome if it disrupts you enough to trigger wrenching gut symptoms. Your best defense against those symptoms is an understanding of the dynamics of gut reactions. Then you can act rapidly to adjust to the changes in your life, minimize their bad effects, and regain your balance so you can go on with important activities.

It's easy to understand how unhappy events such as the loss of your job, divorce, or a death in the family can throw you into spasms. But you will have less pain if you acknowledge your sorrow. Grief at these times is normal and should not be repressed. The person who suffers most is the one who won't allow himself a "good cry."

Perhaps the most heart-wrenching example of this inappropriate "stiff upper lip" attitude came out in my office just a few months ago. I got a visit from another doctor, a heart specialist who had lost his three-year-old daughter in an accident. The toddler was skipping alongside her daddy in the parking lot of a shopping mall. It was dusk, the doctor's arms were full of grocery bags so he wasn't holding his daughter's hand, and weary commuters were darting through the parking lot, making shortcuts home. One of those commuters didn't see the curly-haired child, and crushed her with his automobile. She died before her physician-father could even drop his groceries.

There must have been hundreds of people at the little girl's funeral. I remember howls of grief from the mother and grandparents, and a chorus of sobs, sighs, and sniffles from friends and relatives. It seemed to me that everyone displayed grief except the father. He sat dry-eyed and erect, keeping the same dignified composure I had seen in professional meetings and consultations, and in the operating room. He comforted his wife, and moved gracefully through the crowd thanking friends for their sympathy. He nodded at me, and I must admit I felt silly; I was weeping, but he wasn't.

Later he told me that his weeping could wait no longer. Shortly after the child was buried he began to vomit after each meal. Soon his appetite vanished. He dropped weight, became gaunt and sallow-looking, and finally became too weak to take adequate care of his patients. That's when he came to me. At first, he said, he suspected cancer. But tests ruled that out, and after a while my doctor friend admitted, "I wish I could just go on the top of a mountain somewhere, where nobody would hear me, and scream and scream and scream."

My heart went out to this anguished man, who thought he'd lose his dignity if he wept openly for his dead child. He had to go away, he said, to show his grief. We both agreed that since no organic disease showed up on any of the tests, the vomiting was probably his substitute for screaming. It still plagues him, but our talks have helped, I think. He's gaining back some of his weight.

I think my friend should have taken advantage of the permissive atmosphere of his daughter's funeral to let out at least some of his grief. I find that the rituals of religion that are present in an event such as a funeral are most helpful at these times of crisis. Patients who follow through with complete death ceremonies, such as an elaborate preparation, burial, and grief period, have the least gut trouble as they go through a death crisis. The rituals help because they provide a specified place and time where weeping, hand-wringing, and openly asking for help is expected and appropriate. These feelings can and should come out whether you've lost a loved one or a job, or gotten some other bad news. Funerals are one place for the expression of grief; quiet talks at home with friends and family over other kinds of losses are another place where you should be willing to "let go" and express yourself. I'm not advocating you go overboard. Hysteria is never helpful. But you should be aware that any loss, real or imagined, brings on a sense of grief that cannot be swept away with a brave smile. If you try to pretend you're not affected, you're inviting your sorrow and pain to erupt in the form of gut reactions.

Organic illness can also trigger gut reactions. Anything from a severe cold to a broken leg can upset you enough to bring on gastrointestinal symptoms, and the resulting combination of discomforts often magnifies and prolongs the original disorder. Any type of infectious gastroenteritis is usually worse in the gut reactor, and a virus that would just make a "normal" patient weak or dizzy can bring severe cramping and excessive vomiting to a person with a sensitive gastrointestinal tract. Some foods or food additives that might bring about mild gas or bloating in nongut-reacting patients can cause major problems for the gut reactor. If a gut reactor has a heart attack, cancer, or other serious disorder, he is more likely than other patients to react with poor physical defense mechanisms to that disorder, and to become so upset that his gastrointestinal tract, too, ceases to function properly. Gut reactors with gallstones or gallbladder disease experience more pain and vomiting than do other patients. In short, gut reactors are usually people who are more sensitive physically and more likely to have a hard time overcoming the effects of organic diseases. That's one reason I'm so careful to expose my gut-reacting patients to an intensive physical exam. The unwelcome visit of even a mild organic disease might "unbalance" a gut reactor and cause spasms, but the spasms may, in turn, exist along with some hidden ulcer or internal wound. In any event, illness is one life change that causes stress, and, even if it is only temporary, it can be a signal for the onset of gastrointestinal symptoms.

Happy events can also trigger gastrointestinal symptoms, because these events mean a change in life-style. Planned pregnancy, which is usually a much-desired and happy event, is a prime example. Excessive vomiting in early pregnancy can be a gut reaction, as well as gas and abdominal pain in the later months. Postpartum depression, or the well-known "baby blues," is often accompanied by heartburn and gut spasms. A new father is almost as susceptible to this as is the new and happy but confused mother.

Holidays are also prime-time for gut reactions. Patients pour into my office just before Thanksgiving, Christmas, Hanukkah, Easter, or Passover, all shaken in one way or another by the temporary changes brought about by the holidays. These supposedly happy holidays can affect people in two unpleasant ways. First, they make you think that you should be carefree and thrilled because everything on television, in the shopping malls, and in the newspaper and magazine advertisements stresses the fun and family orientation of holidays. So if life is less than perfect for you at the holiday time, you feel guilty. It's hard for even the most well-balanced family person not to feel lonely or deprived when television advertisements continually project images of grinning grandparents awaiting their family's arrival by the hearth, or adorable toddlers snuggling in their elders' laps to chew on a turkey leg. Suppose you just lost your grandfather? Suppose you don't have a toddler in the house? That's enough to make a susceptible person feel some churning in his guts.

Holidays also bring back childhood memories. If the memories are good and you recall laughter, games, kisses, presents, and tables heaped with food, you might be depressed because you don't have those things in the same way right now. If the memories are bad, and filled with feelings of anger, deprivation, poverty, hunger, loneliness, or family disruption, you might feel a surge of those same emotions now, no matter how wonderful life is for you at the moment. In both cases your memories stir anxiety, which comes out in the form of gut reactions. One patient even expressed it overtly by telling me, "There's no way I can win. I'd just as soon get cramps and go to bed until the holiday is over."

But there is a way you can win. You must recognize the difference between past and present, and between fantasy and reality. You can't change your childhood; that's history. But you can remind yourself that what happened long ago needn't be measured against what's happening now. You can't change holiday advertisements, unfortunately, but you can change the way they affect you. Keep away from those foolish, overidealized, consumer-oriented images as much as possible. When you can't duck the television or radio advertisements, for example, treated as you would a cartoon. Tell yourself it's amusing, but far removed from reality. Don't let anybody tell you how things *should* be, making you feel bad because your lifestyle doesn't conform. Then, enjoy your holiday in a way that suits you best. One physician-friend of mine told me his most unpleasant "holiday" is New Year's Eve. He recalls the awkward moment when the clock struck twelve every year of his early adulthood, and he imagined lovers all over the world stopping to kiss one another. "Trouble is," he sighed, "that I had no one to kiss." Years later, when he was happily married, he still felt bad at the magic moment on New Year's Eve. So he decided to escape from what he calls the "I've-got-to-be-happy" pressure on New Year's Eve by going to a movie. When the late show is over, it's mercifully past midnight.

Individualized holidays such as vacations often bring the same stresses, especially if they involve travel. The planning, shopping, and other preparations, combined with the expenses of travel, are all intensely stressful. This happens even if you're finally realizing your "dream" vacation. Sometimes it's precisely that dream touching off your gut reactions, because your expectations are so high that any problem, even one as minor as a snappy waiter at your hotel restaurant, can cause anxiety significant enough to erupt in your guts.

A forty-two-year-old engineer, who has been my patient for seven years, recently made a bad decision about how to spend his three-week annual leave and paid the price of three weeks of bloating, distention, and diarrhea. He rented a large mobile camper, piled into it with his wife, twin eight-year-old boys and twelve-year-old daughter, and took off for what he hoped would be a scenic tour of the West. What happened?

"The boys were restless and jumpy, cramped into the camper," said my patient. "My daughter cried for her friends. My wife got car-sick a lot, and admitted she'd have rather stayed at a resort hotel. I hated all that driving and I found out you can't force family togetherness. I got so nervous and frazzled from hearing everybody's complaints and whining that it seems all I saw for three weeks was the inside of the camper's little toilet room."

When he finally got home, returned the camper, and settled into his ordinary routine, this gut reactor's diarrhea gradually subsided. It was at least a month, however, before he "felt the churning stop." He still suspects he picked up a virus on the trip, and that it, not his emotions, caused his gastrointestinal symptoms. But I think I'll remind him to select a low-key vacation next year, perhaps at a relaxed beach resort. People like this engineer should avoid traveling from spot to spot on a vacation. If you're a gut reactor, when you reach your vacation destination, stay put.

Travel is hard on everyone, including gut reactors. Chemical changes in water, time changes, bacteria in uncommon or unclean foods, or the body's exposure to unfamiliar viruses often bring about organic gastrointestinal problems. These organic, or "real" disturbances can precipitate functional, or "gut reaction" symptoms. They can also prolong them, and make them much worse. Again, your best defense is a commonsense routine, some simple precautions such as avoiding contaminated water or food, and a realistic expectation that the vacation probably won't all be a bed of roses. If you expect some thorns, they won't hurt as badly.

Another major change stems from your job or career. Ongoing job frustration requires a permanent change, and nothing short of quitting or otherwise drastically altering the situation will help. Gut reactors who are bored, frightened, threatened, or otherwise exposed to job-related stress almost always get sick on their way to the office or factory, while they're there, or even while they're discussing or thinking about the problem.

Other types of illness have also been attributed to job stress. *The New York Times* reported on February 3, 1980, that assembly-line operators got dizzy and nauseous when the pace of their jobs changed, and that work stress was a precipitating factor in ulcers, respiratory disease, angina, and even skin rashes among rubber and chemical-plant employees. One physician quoted in the *Times* article, Dr. Michael J. Colligan, noted that job stress hits at all levels, from the janitor to the top executive. Dr. Colligan, a research psychologist with the National Institute of Occupational Safety and Health, said, "The formation of ulcers in executives has long been a stereotype. But we have found that ulcerization is not exclusively a problem of executives or white collar workers. Now researchers are looking increasingly at workers on assembly lines."

Ulcers are, of course, an organic gastrointestinal disease. But I have found, in my own patients, that people with ulcers usually have gut reactions too. I don't think they necessarily go together and I don't believe, as some doctors do, that gut reactions are a forerunner of ulcers. But patients with sensitive gastrointestinal tracts often exhibit both problems—ulcers and gut spasms—and I check carefully for ulcers both in the stomach and colon when I examine gut reactors.

Some employers, such as the giant Lockheed Corporation, are recognizing the relationship between job stress and illness and are instituting exercise and relaxation programs. That may work for some people, but most patients who are in what they perceive as dead-end jobs must change, or suffer gut symptoms.

The job change itself can easily precipitate gastrointestinal trouble. An involuntary change, such as being demoted or fired, is obviously stress-inducing and is a setup for gut reactions. The best coping mechanism for this type of change is to express your grief to your spouse, clergyperson, doctor, and friends and then quickly find a job that suits you better. A voluntary or welcome change, such as a promotion or a sudden success, is also stressful. You might be worried about meeting new responsibilities, fulfilling added obligations, or living up to your starlike reputation.

Long ago, when I was a medical officer in the army, a young sergeant with alarming gut symptoms came to me. He was vomiting, losing weight rapidly, and suffering constipation followed by urgent, forceful diarrhea. Once or twice he got so dizzy he actually toppled from his chair, and one time he chipped his tooth on the edge of the desk as he fell.

I put him in the infirmary at once. The poor

fellow went through exhausting X-ray and lab tests, and we were both puzzled when they all came back negative. One evening, after work, I dragged a card table to the side of his bed and we began playing poker. We chatted as we played, and the sergeant told me he was "terrified" of his recent promotion to Officer's Candidate School. He hated the desk work, the managerial responsibilities, and the task of supervising large groups of other men. He'd rather be a sergeant, he said, and "Do the work myself, even if it is scut work, because when I do it myself, I know it gets done."

The sergeant eventually got out of the infirmary, finished his schooling, and started his new officer-status job. He lasted at it for a little over a year, then quit the army and went home to work on his father's dairy farm. Years later, I thought about this man whenever I treated a patient whose gut symptoms happened to coincide with a promotion and the assumption of new power and responsibilities on the job. Now I know that some sensitive people simply aren't cut out for the intensity of high-stress, job-related responsibilities. They must be brave enough to turn down promotions and transfers if they are happy where they are. Or if they accept a new workload and suffer too badly from gut symptoms as a result, they should do what my army friend had to do: quit.

Quitting your job is a drastic remedy. What else can you do? Again, don't keep your anxieties to yourself. Tell family and friends you're worried, and don't expect to accomplish everything at once. If you do change your job, accept the new career gradually, as a natural part of life. If you can't or won't change, stop spinning your wheels and find other interests to make your off-job hours more rewarding.

One change becoming more and more "natural" to many people is a rapid shift in family relationships as a result of marriage and divorce. Getting married, no matter how joyful, is an event bristling with possibilities for gut reactions. When you get married you are formalizing a financial, emotional, and sexual commitment to another person. You're saying "I do" to a new home, new friends, new drains on your pocketbook, and a radically altered life-style. There is often an elaborate ceremony to go through, and many times the person getting married is assaulted by friends and relatives who want to give advice or find some other way to interfere with the plans. I sympathize with gut reactors who stick to simple ceremonies to avoid the stress attending every wedding. People get stomachaches at their own weddings whether they're being married for the first or the fourth time.

Divorce is a major change in life-style and can produce acute functional gastrointestinal distress. Most often, the pain comes before the divorce, while the complaining partner is thinking about and planning for the big move. Some people need almost constant medical care while they wrestle with the guilt, fear, and apprehension that precede a divorce. I've noticed once the marriage is finally and formally severed, however, gut symptoms usually ease up considerably. Perhaps it's the agony of making a decision about divorce that causes most of the turmoil. Once the decision is made, the gut reactor seems to feel relieved, and is better able to get an apartment, care for the children, select new furniture, start dating again, and follow through with other tasks which come after a divorce.

"I was so bloated and weak in the six months before my divorce that some days I could hardly move," a thirty-nine-year-old public school administrator told me. "My husband seemed to want a divorce too, but it was mostly up to me to make the break. We were just fighting about everything all the time, and I felt there was no love left at all. Still it was hard; we'd been married 18 years. All the time I was thinking seriously about divorce, I was having terrible stomach problems, mostly bloating. I felt like a balloon, and I knew it was real because I couldn't button the waistband on my skirt, even though I lost twelve pounds.

"When the divorce finally went through, it was like someone pricked me with a pin and my stomach deflated. I could eat and sleep much better. I'm still nervous, of course, because there's a lot going on, a lot to adjust to. I have a new job, we're fighting over alimony, and one of my children is reacting very poorly and flunking school. Still, I'm not overwhelmed, like I was before the divorce, and I definitely don't feel the same bloating."

Gut reactors who take the time to understand their disease are rarely overwhelmed by anything. They can cope with symptoms that might erupt during times of trouble, because they know the temporary nature of the symptoms and aren't afraid they've got an organic illness. And gut reactors who accept their own limitations learn to find success within their careers and personal lives without exposing themselves to more stress than they know they can handle.

I must say once again it is the patient's responsibility to find out as much as he can about his own gut reactions and to decide just how much strain he can take before they erupt. There is simply no substitute for self-awareness. It is your responsibility to equip yourself with the intellectual data leading to emotional acceptance and control of your gut reactions. Your doctor can explain, but he can't listen for you. He can be sympathetic but he can't express your emotions. He can suggest changes in life-style but he can't follow through and actually accomplish these changes. He can recommend ways to handle times of trouble, but you, not the doctor, must adjust to the actual experience. All of this is up to you. Don't be afraid or ashamed to admit openly, to yourself and to others, that times of trouble have stirred anxiety and gut symptoms. Most of us know and accept that concept. Dr. Eddy Palmer, whom I consider one of this nation's outstanding gastroenterologists, said long ago "any situation that creates emotional stimulation can cause pain."

The stimulation of new and/or unexpected life-altering events is necessary and unavoidable. But it usually won't bring lasting pain if you understand what's going on, and remain flexible enough to bend with life's brisk winds.

10

The Rest of Your Life

By now you know that gut reactions are complicated, elusive, and frustrating. Doctors have a hard time categorizing the disorder because it hovers somewhere between the fields of physical and emotional medicine. They even have difficulty naming it. Your problem may be called "functional gastrointestinal disease," "unruly guts," "spastic colon," "irritable bowel," or a number of other things. Even the patient who suffers from one or several symptoms is challenged to describe what he's feeling because these symptoms change, shift, disappear, then pop up again at what seems to be a totally unexpected moment. For some people the symptoms are chronic and ongoing, and they may have been battling them since childhood. For others, gut reactions may be sporadic, coming only when stress hits hard.

It's confusing. How can you control and live with this disorder? What are the prospects for an eventual "cure"? How can you minimize the effects of gut reactions for the rest of your life?

First, you should know that nobody is recorded in modern medical records as dying of gut reactions and nobody, to my knowledge, has had his or her life shortened by the symptoms. Perhaps this is one reason research on the subject is so sparse and slow. Scientists tend to concentrate their best efforts on life-threatening organic problems, such as cancer or heart disease.

As late as September, 1978, according to an article in *The Lancet* which was prepared with the help of thirty-five gastroenterologists, it was admitted that science in general is somewhat at a standstill in the exploration of functional gut problems. The article, "Management of the Irritable Bowel," said all a doctor could do after making a proper diagnosis was reassure his patient that the symptoms, though real enough, "arise not from organic disease such as cancer of the bowel, but from a disorder of function, similar to migraine or asthma." As for future management, the article stated, "If anxiety or depression with an associated irritable-bowel syndrome results from a 'one-of' life event, such as bereavement, medicines may be best avoided in the first instance, with explanation, instead, of the normality of such a reaction.. . ." The article added that switching to a high-fiber diet is sometimes helpful, and drugs do the trick once in a while. Now and then physicians see gut reactors for a long time, and refer stubborn cases to a psychiatrist, said the article, but "Another approach is to admit to the imperfections of even the best medical treatment and encourage the patient, in as helpful and positive a way as possible, to accept and live with the idiosyncrasies and vicissitudes of his intestinal tract."

This shrugging attitude may be one reason research on gut reactions is minimal: doctors may not see much hope for a medical cure. They could be right. I think hope is in another direction. In "Digestive Disease," an article in *Drug Therapy* journal in February, 1980, Doctors Thomas P. Almy and Herbert L. Bonkowsky say that while the science and practice of organic gastroenterology has made progress in the last decade, "in contrast, the understanding and management of functional disorders of the bowel have changed very little in recent years." These doctors add, however, even if functional gut disorders "have been largely ignored by the psychiatrist and gastroenterologist," the outlook for more research in the 80s is bright. Why? Because more people now understand and accept the direct relationship between the human brain and digestive system. I agree.

But if little research is going on right now, how can we be hopeful about controlling gut reactions? Part of the answer is in what Doctors Almy and Bonkowsky say: gut symptoms are increasingly better understood these days. And part of the answer is in what I believe to be a relatively new but overwhelmingly important trend in medicine— the concept that the patient, and not the doctor, is mainly responsible for the maintenance of good health.

For the rest of your life, you'll be aware of your own susceptibility to gut symptoms and your own ultimate responsibility in their management and control. Let me emphasize again that when I refer to gut reactions it would be inappropriate to use the word "cure" except with those telltale quote marks around it. This indicates my belief that while with hard work you can look forward to little or no trouble with your guts in the future, you may never be totally symptom-free, or "cured."

Because of this inability to talk in terms of a "cure," you may be left dangling on the horns of a constant medical dilemma. Almost always, when the symptoms appear for any length of time, you'll have to return to your doctor for a medical evaluation, to make sure no significant organic disease is presenting itself. At the same time, you'll be struggling to avoid an overdependence on the physician and his chemicals, because he and they have a limited role to play in your future management of gut symptoms. The physician's major contribution is diagnosis; his job is to tell the difference between gut reactions and organic disease, and perhaps guide you in achieving mastery over the symptoms. The person primarily responsible for that ultimate mastery, however, is you.

I believe the next big step in dealing with functional gastroenterological disease, and perhaps with all functional diseases, will be made by patients, not doctors. One reason for this is cost: medicine is becoming so expensive that patients will insist on learning more about how to care for themselves, in order to avoid unnecessary office visits, laboratory tests, and prescriptions. Perhaps this is one unexpected but really beneficial effect of inflation. As far as I'm concerned, it's about time patients took more interest in medical information. And, as people become better educated about medicine, they will see their doctors less and less as "miracle men," and more and more as highly-trained but imperfect human beings, who are capable of greed, inefficiency and mistakes. The old concept of the doctor as God will fade away and doctors can breathe a little easier as the terrible burden of exclusive health care is lifted from their shoulders. Patients will, however, probably always reserve a special place in their hearts for the man or woman they see as able to take away pain or who successfully guides them through a terrible illness. Doctors have always had a great deal of power in American society, because, as Dr. George A. Silver put it in *A Spy In the House of Medicine*, "The doctor with his knowledge and skills is a barrier to death and a hopeful warrior on behalf of the sick person. In that context the physician will probably always be respected above others."

We doctors can keep some of this respect and still push people to take care of themselves. Gut reactors should probably lead the way in this new consumer-oriented, take-care-of-yourself movement, because they are in a class by themselves: they need medical care, but they're not really sick. So a gut reactor is in a perfect position to step forward and offer to become a peer and a partner with a physician, with the understanding that he is ready and willing to assume the major responsibility for his own body.

There are some scientists and physicians who believe the patient carries not only the responsibility and capability for his own cure, but the responsibility for his disease as well. Dr. David E. Bresler, director of the Pain Control Unit at the

University of California in Los Angeles, says people with chronic back pain who allow themselves to be made miserable by that pain are suffering because of their mixed-up attitudes toward life. "Almost always," says Dr. Bresler, "people who have chronic pain are also depressed. It's not just their lower back that hurts; their life hurts, and they have placed that hurt in their lower back."

Some cancer and heart specialists are now beginning to suspect that victims of these diseases might be *allowing* the disease to overtake the body, and they say patients who fight back are sometimes remarkably successful.

Not *all* doctors would agree, but medicine in general seems more receptive now to the notion that illness, at least to some extent, is a product of your state of mind. This information was dug up by reporter David Black, who brought it together in an excellent article in a national magazine in April, 1980. The article explored why some people get sick and others don't. It suggested that sad people get sick, and happy people don't. Mr. Black made a rather direct connection between stress and illness, and included in the article a little story about himself which seems particularly appropriate here. He said the article, which involved numerous interviews and a great deal of research, was a major challenge for him and "involved more work than I had ever done before for a single piece." Soon after he started the work, said Mr. Black, he developed "excruciating stomach pains."

"No matter how little I ate, I felt bloated," he said. "I was nauseated 24 hours a day. A few days before ending the research, I happened to be describing my physical symptoms to one of the doctors I was interviewing and apparently coincidentally, mentioned how much trouble I was having digesting all the material I had been gathering.

"He smiled."

" 'Oh, yes; digesting the material,' " the doctor said.

"My body was telling me in a very graphic way—virtually using a physical pun—just that," Mr. Black realized, recognizing his own responsibility for the stomach pains. I think the rest of us, patients and physicians alike, would be wise to do the same.

Putting the spotlight on the patient as the responsible party in any doctor–patient relationship is a fairly new idea. Many doctors may not like this concept, because it pulls away their glittering masks as mystical, potent healers. Many patients may not like it because it burdens them with new and complicated duties and implies that if they become sick because of emotional attitudes or because they don't stick to adequate routine health-care programs, they have only themselves to blame.

There are leading physicians in this country, however, who see this new health movement as part of a larger emphasis on individual responsibility in society. The late Dr. John H. Knowles summarized this concept in December, 1977, in an editorial called "Responsibility for Health" in *Science*. Dr. Knowles, who was president of the Rockefeller Foundation when he wrote the editorial, said "If he is willing to follow reasonable rules for healthy living, [the patient] can extend his life and enhance his own and the nation's productivity. If he is willing to reassert his authority with his children, he can provide for their optimal physical and mental development.'' What we learn from Dr. Knowles is that adults have the potential and the duty to take charge of their own lives, and if they do so successfully, the positive impact of this self-assertion will be felt by their own children and by society at large.

Dr. Knowles went further than simply stating that in order to stay well, a person must give up overeating, smoking, taking pills, and other ''bad habits which many people enjoy.'' He challenged patients to read and learn more about medicine, insist on a larger social and financial investment in fundamental and applied research, and openly challenge the misleading advertisements of many pharmaceutical companies. As far as I'm concerned, gut reactors should be first to accept such a challenge, because they have the most to gain from taking the lead in being well-informed, discriminating medical consumers.

Part of being well-informed on medical issues is knowing that while research on functional gut disorders may be painfully slow right now, progress is being made every day in exploring how stress affects the human body. Doctors Almy and Bonkowsky acknowledge that this progress is bound to have some positive effect in the way we view gut reactions.

''In our view,'' say the doctors, ''the stage is set for several new approaches to controlling functional disorders of the gut or more properly, the psychosocial factors underlying these disorders.

Both curative and preventive benefits may be realized from family counseling, behavior modification, and biofeedback. Extension of the methods of psycho-pharmacology to the visceral brain may be highly effective. Considering that functional disorders represent by far the most common form of gastrointestinal illness in the United States, entailing large expenditures for health services, heavy use of health care resources, and major loss of economic productivity, the pursuit of these research goals should bring welcome social benefits."

To me, the most promising areas for the future control of gut reactions are interview therapy, hypnosis, and biofeedback. I'd like to see more research in all three fields.

Interview therapy is a simple method used by a doctor to allow his gut-reacting patient to express feelings. The "interview" is an exchange between patient and physician, and the patient is encouraged to do most of the talking. The doctor, or interviewer, asks a few general questions that are really invitations to "let it all out." The doctor might gently say, "Tell me how you feel," then sit back and quietly listen as the patient vents his fears, anxieties, or even his hostilities. This is not a physician's attempt at playing analyst; it's his way of allowing the patient to communicate without interruption. In the process, the patient may teach both the doctor and himself a lot about his own hidden emotional responses to his physical distress. The doctor expresses no opinions, offers no solutions, makes no comments, and gives no support; he just listens. Now and then, if the patient rambles or gets off the topic the doctor has to guide the interview and identify areas of discussion. For the most part, however, the doctor is passive.

It's amazing how many patients, after anywhere from five to thirty minutes of interview therapy, tell me, "This is the first time I can remember that anybody, including a doctor, really *listened* to me." Almost without exception, patients who are gut reactors respond well to such therapy and leave my office feeling better. Perhaps they just needed an outlet for their repressed emotions, and the act of "talking out" those emotions served as enough release to ease the symptoms. After about ten hours of this kind of release, I notice a definite overall improvement in gut-reacting patients. And I also notice that if they *don't* get better after ten hours, they probably can't benefit from interview therapy, and it's time to try something else.

There are three kinds of patients who block interview therapy, and for whom it usually won't work at all. Some patients just won't talk. Others talk too much: they chat about their kids, their pets, the weather, or the latest fashions. Their purpose is to evade the task at hand, seemingly by boring the doctor until he ends the session. And some patients just deny their pain and problems and insist everything is really fine.

With patients like this, for whom talking is either too painful or threatening, hypnosis might be helpful.

I don't practice hypnosis. It takes a lot of training, skill, and time to master the techniques of this delicate art, and not many physicians have the interest or ability to make the investment. If I think a patient would benefit from hypnosis, I'll recommend someone I know who has the proper training and who can be trusted to use it in the best way possible. There's a lot of hocus-pocus swirling around the subject of hypnosis, and many patients can't refrain from snickering when I suggest giving it a try. Perhaps they are right in being cautious; some hypnotists bone up on a few techniques, set themselves up in fancy offices, and try to dazzle their customers with claims of immediate cures. Usually, however, a hypnotist who is recommended by a reputable physician is reputable too, and won't offer much in the way of on-the-spot relief. As with everything else, any relief you get by being hypnotized is something you'll have to work for and achieve on your own, with aid and guidance from the hypnotist. And you have to very much want that relief, because contrary to what still might be popular opinion, hypnosis can't make you do anything you don't want to do. It's simply a method of letting you put aside fears that might be blocking your own ability to overcome some of life's problems. In this case, the problems are being manifested in your guts.

Only about seventy percent of the population can be hypnotized and of these not everyone will be helped by the process. Gut reactors, who are acting out their feelings through their gastrointestinal tracts, tend to be "suggestible" or somewhat open to hypnosis. If they are also motivated to rid themselves of one or more gut symptoms, hypnosis could be very helpful.

Another promising area, both right now and for future research in the field of psychosomatic gastroenterology, is biofeedback. Biofeedback is both a theory and a technique. Reduced to its simplest terms, it means the body (bio) can be influenced by the brain and can cause a measurable change in heart rate, blood pressure, muscle spasm, and other so-called involuntary reflexes. The change is measured by a machine, which "feeds back" the information to the patient and doctor. While the doctor interprets the change and encourages the patient to keep trying, the patient uses the feedback to gauge his own progress. For example, if a patient with high blood pressure is hooked up to a biofeedback machine, he can concentrate on lowering the pressure and the machine will show him, perhaps by means of a needle going up or down, whether or not he's doing the job. Being able to see the results of your own efforts on a machine is most encouraging, and biofeedback has been used recently to regulate bodily organs, decrease pain, and even help a paralyzed woman emerge from her bed and sit up straight. Experiments are now going on to enable people to do biofeedback without a machine; this is called autogenic training.

Biofeedback depends, to a great extent, on trial and error, and in that way is similar to all forms of learning. The patient is learning how to regulate his own bodily functions. Dr. Marvin M. Schuster, professor of medicine and assistant professor of psychiatry at Johns Hopkins School of Medicine in Maryland, has used biofeedback to combat a variety of gastrointestinal problems. Dr. Schuster says it's too early to tell if this technique will be one answer to getting rid of gut reactions, but so far he's enthusiastic about his results. He has demonstrated that patients with irritable bowel symptoms can learn to suppress their abnormal gut contractions with biofeedback. Patients with severe fecal incontinence, for example, who could not control their bowel movements, have learned through biofeedback how to increase or relax the pressure in their lower colons so they could lead normal lives again. Patients who suffered from reflux, or severe heartburn when partly digested food leaped back up instead of down their throats, managed to tighten their esophageal sphincters by using biofeedback, thus eliminating the problem. Before we had biofeedback, both these feats were thought to be impossible, because doctors believed that they were "involuntary" bodily functions. This meant they were beyond our control. Dr. Schuster and others, however, have shown that we humans have control over a lot of what goes on in our bodies—perhaps more than we ever dreamed possible. It may not be too much to think that some day we might be able to regulate the ticking of our own hearts. Certainly, the regulation of our guts is a reasonable goal.

Patients who want to try biofeedback are referred to experts in the field who set up certain criteria to determine which patients will be accepted for treatment. The patient must be motivated, and have a strong desire to rid himself of his handicap, whether it's paralysis, gut reactions, or something else. Next, the patient must be aware of the desired response—a lessening of stomach pain, for example—and be able to feel that response. After that, the patient has to be able to influence the response; he has to be able to concentrate enough to actually make the response happen. Finally, the patient must read and appreciate the feedback so he'll go on to even greater levels of achievement. According to Dr. Schuster, about two-thirds of the patients who meet these conditions can learn to control their gut symptoms in about ten biofeedback sessions. Some people get much better after about three sessions, and all of the patients who improve keep that improvement as a long-term result of the biofeedback process.

I'm certain that a lot of exciting new developments are just around the corner in controlling gut reactions through interview therapy, hypnosis, and biofeedback. And I'm just as certain that diet and drugs will prove to be less and less important.

The only real step forward we've made in connecting overall diet to any improvement in functional gastrointestinal disorders is in the regular and consistent use of high-bulk foods. Even though various "easy-going" diets have been used extensively by doctors and patients in an attempt to calm unruly guts, and even though I've often experimented with diet myself for the benefit of certain patients, there is very little solid evidence to say that it makes any sense. Many gut reactors still put great faith in bland diets, avoid coffee and chocolate, or turn away from salads. However, as early as 1969, Dr. R. H. Salter, a gastroenterologist in Bristol, England, disputed the use of diet for patients with gut symptoms. In his article in the *Lancet*, "What Should the Patient Eat?" Dr. Salter said: "Most diets are unpleasant, expensive, difficult to adhere to, tedious to prepare and cause considerable inconvenience to the patient and to his relatives." Worse than that, said Dr. Salter, diets usually don't work.

Like almost everybody else in American society, gut reactors are confused about what they should and shouldn't eat. What causes the confusion? Perhaps doctors have failed to give solid advice on the nutritional values of basic foods, and advertisers have stepped in to take advantage of the public's resulting ignorance. Daniel S. Greenberg, who wrote "Nutrition: A Long Wait for a Little Advice," in the February, 1980, issue of *New England Journal of Medicine*, does say that media advertising plays a powerful role in forming Americans' food preferences. If you are bombarded by commercials for a certain food you'll have a hard time resisting when you see it on the grocery store shelf. If you read often enough that beets or cranberries might be bad for you, chances are you'll eliminate them from your diet without ever investigating the source of the reports. The best way to decide on your own diet is to learn as much as you can about basic nutrition (ask your doctor, or get books and research materials on his recommendation) and plan your daily menus around foods that are wholesome and pleasing to you. As a general rule, fresh foods are best and canned or processed foods offer little nutritional value. But it's the processed foods which get the most attention in television and newspaper advertisements. The processed food lobby is wealthy and powerful, and so far all doctors can do is to educate themselves and their patients individually and back up their plugs for fresh foods with a reference to books like *Healthy People,* published by the U.S. Public Health Service. The book says, "Food advertising, particularly on television, has a powerful influence on food choices. Many foods are promoted for their convenience and easy preparation or for the taste rather than for nutritional value. Convenience and good taste are important considerations, but a balanced presentation should also consider nutritional value.''

My point is that gut reactors need the same good foods as other healthy, normal people, and for the most part should not try for anything more than nutrition when they select what goes into their mouths. Gut reactors don't need special diets of any sort, and should make a point of staying well-informed about nutrition. A healthy diet will help keep you in good shape generally, and thus make you better able to concentrate on fighting your disorder in other, more fruitful directions.

Except for their stress on high-bulk foods, wheat, and vegetables, "health food nuts" don't do any better at overcoming gut reactions than people on "normal" diets. "Organic" foods—whatever they may be—are no better or worse for you than nonorganic foods. Dr. Thomas H. Jukes, of the University of California, wrote an article in the *Journal of the American Medical Association* in 1974 called "The Organic Food Myth." In it, he rebukes the organic food industry for falsely claiming that their products cure or prevent disease, and says these claims have no documentation. He says, "I conclude that the majority of the public has been so influenced by erroneous information supplied by the 'health food' movement that the general understanding of nutrition is, for the most part, lost. I have not really seen in the literature, nor experienced in my patients, significant improvement from their functional gastrointestinal symptoms of any sort by the use of 'organic' foods or 'health' food or many of the multitude of special additives, specially processed foods, or by the omission of additives in food.''

If you're a gut reactor who likes nuts, wheat germ, bran, fresh vegetables, fruit and fruit juices, and prefers lean meat and few sweets, and *that's* your idea of "health foods," you're in good shape. If you're insisting on "organically-grown" foods and are obsessed with vitamins, roots, and herbs, and *that's* your idea of health foods, watch out. You're probably wasting your time, your money, and your energies searching for some food-related relief from your symptoms. For now and, I suspect, in the future, that type of search will prove futile.

Hoping for new drugs to ease your symptoms is probably just as futile as hoping for a "cure" through organic foods. I don't see any big future breakthroughs in drugs to help gut reactors. In contrast, I do see big trouble ahead for people who like to use or experiment with drugs to any great extent, because certain drugs can cause or worsen gut symptoms. In an August, 1966, article in *Drug Therapy* medical magazine, two professors at the University of Chicago, Doctors Jeffrey J. Glass and Joseph B. Kirsner, noted that drug-induced gut symptoms are more common than we think. The article, "Drug-induced Gastrointestinal Disease—A Brief Overview," said at least five percent, and perhaps an even greater percentage, of patients who go into the hospital for one reason or another get drugs which throw their digestive systems out of whack.

Drugs cause gut problems in a variety of ways. Some drugs change the way cells react, and thus influence your body's absorption of nutrients. Drugs can influence glandular secretions, change the way your intestines move, or cause inflammation in the gastrointestinal tract that leads to ulceration and bleeding. Drugs also can cause nausea, vomiting, diarrhea, painful spasms, or constipation.

One drug can easily lead to another, putting the patient on a dangerous medical merry-go-round. For example, you might take codeine to ease the pain of your writhing intestines. But this drug causes constipation, and now you're tempted to take a laxative. And laxatives may be among the most abused drugs in the Western world. Some doctors say laxative abuse has reached epidemic proportions. Doctors A. I. Morris and L. A. Turnberg, in their article, "Surreptitious Laxative Abuse," in the 1979 issue of the *Journal of Gastroenterology*, said, "In 1975, in the U.S.A., $130 million was spent on laxatives, and in the United Kingdom, the National Health Service spent £7 million, and probably several times this amount was sold over the counter. Between 15 and 30 percent of the population over the age of 60 take laxatives regularly, and they can choose from among the 700 or so different preparations available in the U.S.A. or the 200 available in the United Kingdom."

Other doctors and I have seen what all this overuse of laxatives, in the hospital and at home, can do. Patients turn up with cramps, diarrhea, metabolic disturbances, and nutritional difficulties, all as a result of taking laxatives. Things aren't likely to get better in the future as far as laxatives and other drugs are concerned, and my best advice to gut reactors is to be stingy and cautious in the use of any drug, and never to take anything without a doctor's thoughtful consent. Even when a drug is prescribed, be sure to ask your doctor what it is, what it does, why he's prescribing it, and what possible side effects you can expect. If you can't get any satisfactory answers, throw away the prescription (and maybe the doctor, too).

The doctor who shouldn't be discarded is the one who will look to the future with you, by teaming up with you as your partner and medical educator in a joint quest for the understanding that will lead to symptomatic relief. To be as free as possible from gut reactions for the rest of your life, you need something more than advances in pure medicine. I believe you need a good relationship, between you and your doctor. To me, a doctor must be more than a well-trained scientist. He or she must also be a caring, sympathetic, hopeful person who is willing to form an almost mystical partnership with a gut-reacting patient. I feel certain that many unexplained "cures" are based on such a partnership.

I'm not alone in thinking future strides in medicine will travel along this sort of human-relations path. In his article, "What Are Physicians For?" in the September, 1977, issue of the *Journal of the American Medical Association*, Dr. Ronald A. Carson of the University of Florida said this sort of thinking has been around for at least fifty years, and good doctors are still striving for a better working relationship with patients. In 1927, Dr. Francis Peabody set down the classic admonition for beginning doctors in his now-famous essay, "The Care of the Patient," which was also published in the *Journal of the American Medical Association*. Dr. Peabody warned, ". . . the essence of the practice of medicine is that it is an intensely personal matter . . . the significance of the intimate personal relationship between physician and patient cannot be too strongly emphasized, for in an extraordinarily large number of cases, both diagnosis and treatment are directly dependent upon it, and the failure of the young physician to establish this relationship accounts for much of his ineffectiveness in the care of patients."

Dr. Carson took note of Dr. Peabody's warnings in his article, and stressed the "intimate personal relationship" as the foundation upon which all patient relief and physician satisfaction is based. One of the oldest meanings of our English word "personal," said Dr. Carson, is "to look upon persons with favor, to respect them, to accept them." And Dr. Carson added that to achieve that personal feeling within the guidelines of a professional relationship, the physician must be interested in all his patients, and listen to them with "an empathetic ear, an ear that hears more than the obvious, and by questioning in a fashion that illicits meaning and perception as well as literal answers."

Another doctor who believes strongly in the patient-physician relationship as a healing agent is Edmund D. Pellegrino, president of the Catholic University of America and professor at Georgetown University. In 1979 Dr. Pellegrino wrote a book on medical philosophy, *Humanism and the Physician*, in which he defines a doctor's compassion.

Compassion is not some facile combination of talents in public relations under the rubric of bedside manner; nor is it some mystical quality of charisma which radiates only from the gifted; nor again is it synonymous with mawkish or demeaning pity for the sick, or a saccharine piety and self-righteousness. These construals [*sic*] are all offensive to true compassion and an insult to the wounded humanity of the patient.

Compassion means to feel genuinely the existential situation of a person who is bearing the burden and who has undergone the insult of sickness to his whole being. We can never enter wholly into the state of being of another human, but we must strive with all our might to *feel* it to the fullest extent our sensibilities will allow. It is our failure to feel along with the patient that leads to the complaint we hear so often today of humiliation and being demeaned.

If by this set of definitions Dr. Pellegrino has set out the future goals of the physician, what can be the future goals of the patient? As a gut reactor these goals are critical to you, because you may be in contact with a physician for long-term care that will determine the course of your life.

Your goals should be (1) being able to relate your personality and emotions to gut symptoms; (2) understanding your body and your disease, and feeling secure in this knowledge; (3) trusting your doctor to help you tell the difference between organic and functional disease; (4) being able to find and stick with the doctor who's right for you; (5) understanding specific symptoms and how you can control them; (6) realizing how your relationships to family and friends interact with gut reactions, and how you can affect these people with or because of the symptoms; (7) little or no reliance on diet and drugs; (8) a healthy overall life-style; (9) ability to cope with change and; (10) a full realization and acceptance that responsibility for a better future rests mainly with you.

These goals basically sum up the ten chapters of this book. Working toward them means you got our essential message: that while gut reactions may be your symptom, they are not your fate. Gut reactors have a lot of work to do, but they have a lot working for them, too, and the future is bright. Your goals are within reach, and the rest of your life is up to you.

Glossary

We carry a world—perhaps a universe—within us, in the form of our own bodies. Our hearts pump, our blood surges, our cells live and reproduce and die, and we take it all for granted. No computer works as marvelously as our own brains; no machine is as efficient as our liver; no hinge as perfect as the knob of bone in our knees. Yet what do we know about all this? Very little. Doctors and research scientists have found out a great deal about the chugging factories within us, and their knowledge both comforts and amazes us. But what is really amazing is what they *don't* know. They don't know how a fetus is formed, or what the function is (or ever was) of the appendix. There's an old joke in which doctors try to laugh away their astonishing ignorance: A patient says to his doctor, "If science is answering all the questions of the universe, how is it that you still believe in God?" And the doctor replies, "Because I can't find any other explanation for ear wax."

If doctors confess to a certain amount of ignorance about the human body, then we common folk must indeed be lost souls. And when it comes to our most precious possession—our own physical beings, for which there is no replacement—we usually *are* lost. Biologist Lewis Thomas, president of the Memorial Sloan-Kettering Cancer Center in New York and a well-known scientific essayist (his books, *The Lives of a Cell* and *The Medusa and the Snail*, have both hit the *New York Times* best-seller list), answered some questions about science recently in which he stressed our lack of awareness and knowledge about medicine in general, and our bodies in particular. In the April, 1980, issue of *Smithsonian* magazine, teacher and author Timothy Ferris asked Thomas how far we all had to go in reaching the limits of scientific knowledge, and quoted Thomas' earlier reply, which was, ". . . I cannot begin to guess at all the causes of our cultural sadness, not even the most important ones, but I can think of one thing that is wrong with us and eats away at us: we do not know enough about ourselves. We are ignorant about how we work, about where we fit in, and most of all about the enormous, imponderable system of life in which we are imbedded as working parts. We do not really understand nature, at all . . . We are *dumb*."

Most of us feel that way, even if we won't admit it. We have only one body, and it has only one life. We often spend that life acquiring vast amounts of knowledge about art, music, law, or whatever our particular interest may be, yet we are helpless as infants when asked to point to the spot on our bellies where the appendix is located.

In particular, most of us know very little about our digestive systems, yet we certainly couldn't live without this complex network. Worse than our ignorance, perhaps, is the flood of misinformation that pours our way when we complain about a pain here or a cramp there; everyone loves to spew advice about a possible "cure" for the digestive disorders that might afflict us, even if they know nothing about the organ in question. Dr. Grant Thompson put it bluntly in his book for students and physicians, *The Irritable Gut*. He said, "Man has landed on the moon, conquered smallpox, and explored the secrets of the proton, yet has astonishing ignorance of his own bowels. With the possible exception of the weather, no subject is so prone to uninformed comments."

We can't dispel all that ignorance in this book, partly because we share it. We can't even tell you all we do know about how the digestive system works, because that took years of medical training and experience on David's part, and years of studying science and writing about it from Maxine. But we can share some very basic terms and concepts with you in the form of the following glossary. Please remember this is only a partial and rather unscientific list; we've included only what we thought were the major organs of the digestive tract, major diagnostic procedures, most common operations, medicines, and some medical terminology.

Our hope is that the glossary will make you less bewildered abut what's going on inside your own body.

Major Organs of The Digestive Tract

ANUS: This is the end of the digestive tract. Think of it as a valve, which holds back fecal material until it can be voluntarily defecated. The anus serves as a barrier between the rectum and the outside of your body; without it, you wouldn't be able to control your bowels. Hemorrhoids are located in the anus, but you don't notice them until they get swollen, and hurt.

APPENDIX: This little pouch dangles from the cecum, or first part of the large intestine, and has a nasty habit of getting infected. That seems to be the only way anybody notices the appendix, because it apparently has no function, and if it ever was useful doctors simply don't know about it. Trouble in the appendix is manifested by sharp pains on the right side of the body just below your navel. Surgery usually follows.

COMMON BILE DUCT: This little tube between the liver and the gallbladder allows secretions to flow between the two organs and thus aids in food digestion. When the duct gets blocked by a stone or tumor, the salts, acids, and other dark-colored chemicals that make up bile may back up into your bloodstream. The result is that your skin takes on a darker tone; you become jaundiced.

DUODENUM: This is the first part of the small intestine, where food is absorbed. It is a pinkish, wet tube about ten inches long, and as wide as a small banana. When empty it collapses and lays flat; when filled with food or gas, it expands.

ESOPHAGUS: This soft, pinkish tube, glistening with mucous, starts at the back of your neck and travels down to the stomach. Food slides and is pushed down this tube as you eat, unless you have *dysphagia*, or trouble swallowing. The mucous in the esophagus is a lubricant, which gives this and other internal organs a constantly wet and shiny appearance. Each of your intestinal organs, like the stomach, has specific glands to secret its own mucous. Saliva, for example, is secreted in the mouth and softens and lubricates food for easy swallowing.

GALLBLADDER: Perhaps the only pretty organ inside you is the gallbladder; it's robin-egg blue. That's too bad, because it often gets clogged with stones and has to be surgically removed. The gallbladder is a little bag that pops off the duct between the liver and the small intestine. Its function is to store the bile needed for digestion. When the bile, for some unknown reason, loses its liquid state and becomes solid, a gallstone forms. When the stone (or stones) gets big enough to cause pain, the entire gallbladder is removed. Surgeons have found that just removing the stone will not suffice; usually, another one quickly forms, or the gallbladder, once invaded and then sewn up, can burst. So, it's best to remove the gallbladder. Its function doesn't seem to be an important one for the body, since the unstored bile simply flows through the system, doing its job just as well without a gallbladder. Your gallbladder is located in the right upper abdomen, just below your ribs. It's about the size of a large plum.

GASTROESOPHAGEAL JUNCTION: This is a place, not an organ. It's the area between the esophagus and stomach, right below your breastbone.

HEMORRHOIDS: These are veins in the anus, and as far as we know, they have no crucial function. So, when they become swollen and inflamed, they can be surgically removed if necessary and no harm is done. Other, nearby veins take over the job of removing blood from that tender area.

LIVER: This soft, "squooshy" bag is a complex chemical factory, and you can't live without it. The liver contains hundreds of chemical pathways that perform intricate and interchangeable jobs, all geared toward the disposing of your body's natural and foreign poisons. The liver also secrets digestive enzymes and bile, which go into the intestines. Located just below the lungs and rib cage on the upper right part of your body, the liver is brownish-red in color and weighs about two or three pounds. The liver is most susceptible to hepatitis, which is an inflammation usually caused by a virus, and cirrhosis, which is scarring most often caused by excessive intake of alcohol. If the liver becomes too inflamed or scarred to do its job, the body's poisons accumulate and life ends.

LARGE INTESTINE OR COLON: This bodily "tube" is about four feet long and three inches wide. When filled with feces, it can expand to the width of a kitchen rolling pin. In the large intestine, fluid is drained from residual food and solid feces are formed. This "tube" starts on the right lower side of your body and loops across to the left lower side, so if something goes wrong here you will feel pain almost anywhere in your lower abdomen.

LOWER ESOPHAGEAL SPHINCTER: This is a valve at the junction between your esophagus and stomach. It keeps digested food from coming back up from the stomach into the esophagus, and is regulated by nerves and hormones. When this valve, which is made of muscle and connective tissue, goes awry, food "burps" up the wrong way. The result? You get reflux, or heartburn.

PANCREAS: This organ is located just below your navel and slightly to the left. Its purpose is to secrete digestive enzymes and hormones, the most important of which is insulin. When the pancreas is severely damaged by gallbladder disease, pancreatitis (an inflammation), or heavy alcohol consumption, its function decreases and it often causes severe pains. You might lose your vital supply of insulin, and if so, like a diabetic, you must take it artificially for the rest of your life.

RECTUM: The rectum is the last part of the large intestine. It's about six inches long and can expand to the size of an average man's foot. Its purpose is to store feces until they are evacuated. When empty the rectum is a big, hollow organ; when filled, it can hold a large amount of feces.

SMALL INTESTINE: Two sets of muscles propel food along twenty feet of small intestines in your body, and the process looks like the gyrations of a slow-moving snake. The major acts of digestion take place here. The small intestine is pinkish and wet with mucous, and is about the width of a screwdriver handle. This long organ curls around your entire abdominal cavity, so pain in the small intestine could show up just about anywhere.

STOMACH: Major digestive work is done by this pinkish, shimmering pouch, which is about the size of a shoe box. It receives food and begins to break it down for absorption into the body. When empty, the stomach is like a flat sock; when full, it swells like a medium-sized balloon. As food is digested, the balloon slowly deflates. Your stomach is located on the upper left side of your body, just above the navel. It is, perhaps, the best known of your digestive organs, and people have a tendency to refer to the entire abdominal area as "the stomach."

Major Diagnostic Procedures

When you and your doctor first attack the problem of gut reactions, there is no sure way for either of you to know if the symptoms are stress signals or indications of disease. To be on the safe side you must rule out organic disease before you try to deal with stress. The only way to do this is to go through one or more diagnostic procedures developed to help your doctor explore your gastrointestinal tract and make medical judgments about what he finds there.

All of these procedures take time, and a few are quite expensive. Some of them require lengthy, unpleasant preparations; you'll have to starve for twelve hours before taking one exam, and purge yourself with enemas for another. Some of them are uncomfortable, and a few are so painful that most people need heavy sedation before the exam. None of them are fun.

When your doctor orders a gastrointestinal exam, find out as much as you can about it before you slink into the X-ray room with those silly hospital gowns flapping around your knees. Ask why the exam is being done (what is your doctor looking for?); how much time and money is involved (get specific); where and how it's done (an office exam is better than a hospital outpatient exam because the facilities are usually less unpleasant); what preparation or aftermath is involved, if any (if you're going to be hungry or sore, you'd better know it); who will do the exam (your doctor or a hospital technician); and exactly what you can expect in terms of pain (so you'll know enough to ask for sedation if you're the type who needs it). You should also know that doctors and patients have a different perception of pain. Doctors usually don't like to drug their patients during these procedures; it's expensive and carries an extra risk for the patient. But patients tend to be unable to get their minds off the tube going down their throats or into theic rectums, and their embarrassment and fear often heighten their awareness of discomfort during gastrointestinal exams. Pain perception also differs from patient to patient and depends a lot on your confidence in the skill and swiftness of the doctor doing the procedure.

Like drugs, these procedures should be taken only after you're satisfied they are necessary and you know enough about them to cooperate intelligently. This list will help but for the specifics of your case, ask your doctor.

BARIUM ENEMA: This undignified and sometimes painful procedure is also called a "lower GI series" because it involves a series of X-rays taken of your entire colon.

Its purpose is to look for tumors, infections, ulcers, or narrowing in the colon. To prepare for the exam, you'll need to stay on a liquid diet for about a day beforehand, and take several enemas to clean out your system. The exam takes place in an X-ray room, where barium is injected into the rectum and forced up into the colon. Barium is a white, chalky element that isn't absorbed into the body, so it shows up well on X-rays. It tends to harden and be constipating. The exam takes about thirty minutes and can cause some cramping, so if you're sensitive you may want to ask your doctor for some mild sedation. After the exam, you may feel slightly sore and your feces will be white for at least the rest of the day, as your body expels the barium. You'll probably go skipping out of the X-ray room, however, because you'll be so glad it's over.

COLONOSCOPY: This may be the most painful of all the gastrointestinal diagnostic procedures, and you should insist on adequate sedation before you go through with it. Some doctors do use anesthesia to perform a colonoscopy, but this is an added risk that could keep you in the hospital longer than necessary to do the exam, which ordinarily takes anywhere from fifteen minutes to an hour depending on what the doctor finds. He's looking for abnormalities in the entire colon, and to do this he pushes a tube into your rectum that will give him a first-hand look—not X-rays—of your entire colon. The tube is about 100 inches long and as thick as a man's thumb. As it snakes its way around the colon, air may be forced up the tube to "blow up" this organ and afford the doctor a better view. The tube and air will leave you feeling bloated and sore for at least a day after this exam. You'll have to prepare for it with enemas and diet for a day beforehand, too, so you will be uncomfortable for two or three days. But it's worth a try, because this may be the only way to be sure your colon is healthy, and it may take the place of an exploratory operation.

COMPLETE PHYSICAL EXAM: The touching, feeling, and poking that go on during a complete physical exam is your doctor's most basic diagnostic procedure. It's the only way he can know your body thoroughly, and all the further diagnosis and therapy you receive will be based on this initial exam. A good "physical" should involve your whole body. It includes a careful inspection of your eyes, ears, and throat; listening to your heart and lungs; feeling your abdomen for lumps or swelling; looking at your skin and bone joints for clues to any possible disease; and putting a gloved finger into your rectum to feel for tumors, enlarged prostate in men, or other abnormalities. Even before the doctor does the physical, it should begin with his nurse taking your temperature, pulse, weight, and blood pressure, and possibly include a vision, hearing, and breathing test.

A careful history of your past illnesses and family diseases is important, too, and will bring the time needed for a complete physical exam up to forty-five minutes or an hour. The exam does not include laboratory tests; these will vary from patient to patient, as will any further diagnostic tests.

COMPUTERIZED AXIALTOMOGRAPHY (CT SCAN): The doctors who developed this new and very sophisticated X-ray machine were rightfully awarded the 1980 Nobel Prize for Medicine. The CT scan represents an advance in medicine that can be likened, perhaps, to the discovery of the X-ray itself. With the scan, a patient simply lies on an X-ray table and multiple X-rays "scan" the entire abdomen, showing a full outline of all its internal organs. There is no preparation or pain involved, and the whole thing is over in about forty-five minutes. The scan takes the place of other invasive and painful procedures in many cases, and exposes you to about the same radiation as a barium enema and upper gastrointestinal series. Some medical people have criticized the scan because the machine is so expensive, but it could be cheaper in the long run because it eliminates some hospital stays and many other tests.

ENDOSCOPIC RETROGRADE CHOLANGIOPANCREATOGRAPHY (ERCP): This tongue-twisting diagnostic test involves swallowing a forty-inch-long tube through which the doctor visualizes the tiny ducts of your liver, gallbladder, and pancreas. Through the tube, a dye is injected that outlines the entire organ, so X-rays can be taken. The doctor is looking for tumors, stones, infections, and blockages; X-rays are taken then and there, and a diagnosis can usually be made on the spot. You'll be in the X-ray room for thirty minutes to an hour, and you'll need heavy sedation. You can't be totally "out," because you'll have to move around on the X-ray table as your doctor threads the tube into the ducts, but with enough sedation you shouldn't feel anything. Once this test is finished, you can go home.

GASTROSCOPY or UPPER-GASTROINTESTINAL PANENDOSCOPY: Again, a forty-inch tube about one-half inch thick is swallowed, this time to give the doctor a firsthand look at your esophagus, stomach, and duodenum. Through the tube, which has a light at the end of it, the doctor can see any possible disease of the lining of your upper gastrointestinal tract. You'll be put on a twelve-hour fast before this procedure is done, and given medication to prevent gagging when the tube goes down. Mild sedation is a good idea, too, because few people feel calm about a tube jiggling in their guts, although the sensation is more discomfort than pain. When the tube gets to your stomach, air is forced in to expand this organ for a better look, so you'll feel bloated for a while. The test takes about ten minutes, and there are usually no aftereffects.

LAPAROSCOPY: This test isn't done often, because it requires a doctor with enough skill and experience to cut an inch-long opening in your abdomen and insert a thin tube to look for infections or tumors. The doctor can get a close peek at your liver, spleen, and the lining of your abdomen this way, but the procedure requires a short hospital stay and shouldn't be done without heavy sedation and local anesthesia.

LIVER BIOPSY: If you're jaundiced or the doctor has some other reason to suspect liver disease, he'll order this test. It involves slipping a thin needle into your right side, where the liver is located, and slicing off a piece of this organ so it can be studied in the laboratory. This is called a *percutaneous* or "through the skin" test. You'll lose a piece of liver about one or two inches long and as thick as the lead in an automatic pencil. The whole thing takes only a few minutes but it hurts; you'll need some mild sedation and a local anesthetic. Expect to be sore for a few days, too.

ORAL CHOLECYSTOGRAM: Before you take this painless X-ray exam, you'll swallow iodine pills which, when mixed with your bile, will outline your gallbladder so it will show up nicely. The purpose is to look for gallstones. The X-rays take about ten minutes, and there are no aftereffects.

PERCUTANEOUS CHOLANGIOGRAPHY: This is another "through the skin" test, similar to a liver biopsy. This time, however, the long, thin flexible needle that's stuck into your side carries dye which is injected into the ducts of your liver and gallbladder so these organs can be X-rayed. The procedure is done in the X-ray room, and the X-rays are taken immediately. This procedure takes ten minutes to an hour, depending on the doctor's aim; sometimes it takes more than one jab for the needle to find its exact target. This hurts, so ask for moderate sedation—enough to make you light-headed. You won't be stabbed to death because the needle is flexible. It's called the Chiba needle, and is named after the medical school in Japan where this procedure was perfected.

PROCTOSCOPY-SIGMOIDOSCOPY or PROCTOSIGMOID-OSCOPY: It's too bad that this is an important diagnostic test for anybody with gut symptoms, because it's so undignified. With your head down and your rear end up, you must submit to the insertion of a tube into your rectum, so the doctor can search for polyps, tumors, colitis, or other significant gastrointestinal disease. The tube is about as thick as a fountain pen, and ten inches long. In the hands of a skilled doctor there is no pain, but it doesn't feel great and there may be some bloating if air is used to inflate your rectum so it can be seen better. This test shouldn't take more than three to five minutes, but ask for a tranquilizer if you're the fidgety type.

SMALL BOWEL BIOPSY: This procedure can be done in the doctor's office or as an outpatient in a hospital. It's called a *peroral* or "by the mouth" exam. You must swallow a flexible tube, about one-fourth of an inch wide and forty inches long. The tube is topped by a tiny knife, which pops out when it hits the lining of your upper intestines. A tiny piece of the intestinal lining is sliced off, sucked into the tube, and removed for inspection under a microscope. This doesn't hurt, but the procedure is uncomfortable because the tube makes you gag. Ask for moderate sedation, and expect to spend twenty minutes to an hour with the tube inside you. When it's over, you'll feel too relieved to notice any soreness.

ULTRASONOGRAPHY: Totally painless, this test uses SONAR waves to bounce off your abdomen and detect the presence of tumors or stones, mainly in your gallbladder. It's somewhat like an X-ray except that you are exposed to no radiation, and the only discomfort—it tickles, actually—comes when the technician smears a cold, jellylike substance on your abdomen to keep the SONAR probe in place.

UPPER GASTROINTESTINAL SERIES: This may be the most common of all gastrointestinal diagnostic procedures. To prepare, you'll fast for twelve hours before the exam, then be asked to swallow a "barium milkshake" so your upper intestinal organs will show up on X-rays. This chalky-tasting substance isn't a gourmet's delight, and some desperate doctors have even tried to sweeten the taste with mint. Sometimes that works, but a lot of patients throw up anyway. Once you've got the stuff down, it will zip through your guts quickly, outlining possible tumors, ulcers, and narrowings of the esophagus, stomach, and small intestines. X-rays are taken on the spot, and a radiologist is usually present to watch the barium as it travels. This journey can be seen on a small television screen, so ask the operator to turn it your way so you can watch, too. There's no pain involved, but you should know that barium is constipating so eat a lot of bran after this test.

VENA PUNCTURE: This is a basic blood test which gives your doctor clues about the presence of any infection or tumor in your body. It can also help detect diabetes, gout, leukemia, chemical imbalance, liver malfunction, insufficient internal organ secretions, abnormal blood clotting, poisons, and drugs. To do all this, you'll have to donate from one to four tubes, or about an ounce, of blood. But that has no effect on your body, and if the nurse is skilled, the needle jab in your arm is almost painless. If you get weak at the sight of your own blood, look away while the tube is being filled.

Common Medical Terminology (Mostly to Describe Gastrointestinal Diseases)

Doctors and patients may talk to one another, but too often they are speaking a different language. The patient may appear with symptoms he cannot articulate or explain, and the doctor may not even listen. Instead, he hurriedly scratches out a prescription for an odd-sounding drug, in a handwriting that looks like hieroglyphics, and tosses off an unpronounceable diagnosis when the patient asks, "What's the matter with me?"

Not all doctors do this, of course. Many try their best to communicate with patients, but it takes a lot of time and energy to explain complicated medical facts to a lay person who may be too scared to understand anyway. And, doctors have been conditioned and trained to think in medical jargon; their language really *is* different. Maybe they shouldn't bear the full burden of translating it for patients. Maybe the patient should learn some common medical terms to help the communication process along.

One of the patient's greatest fears is that he or she won't understand what the doctor is saying, and will be too ashamed to ask. Another fear is that the doctor is lying. The patient thinks, "Maybe this doctor is hiding the awful truth from me . . . maybe he's using big words so I won't understand what's going on." Charles Panati, in his 1980 book, *Breakthroughs*, described what he called a "truth box" or miniature voice lie detector which in the future may be plugged into people's telephones to tell them if the person on the other end is fibbing. Many patients, trembling on the telephone, may wish to have a truth box when they talk to their doctors. A "translation box" would help too.

For the time being, however, education will have to take the place of magic boxes. That's the purpose of the following list: to familiarize you with some common medical terms. Once you know them you won't be quite as puzzled by "doctor talk," or quite as intimidated. And you may feel braver about telling your doctor, "I don't understand what you just said. Let's go over it again—together."

ANOREXIA: This means "loss of appetite," and can vary from mild to severe, where the patient refuses all nourishment. Anorexia is usually the first sign of any illness, functional or organic. Total anorexia can last a month or more; that's how long you can survive without solid food, but you can't go for over ten or twelve days without liquids or you'll die of dehydration.

CACHEXIA: When you look like a skeleton and are chronically ill because you're malnourished, you have cachexia. The term describes the loss of a great amount of weight and body mass. It's possible to lose one-half of your weight and survive, although you'd be weak and ill. When weight loss occurs, your body first "eats" its own fat and the muscle and tissue. The major organs like the brain, liver, and kidneys go last.

CANCER, or CARCINOMA: This is the name for any malignancy or uncontrolled growth anywhere in the body. It is dangerous if it spreads from one spot to multiple places and affects vital organs.

CIRRHOSIS: This term means both a disease and the resulting scarring of the liver. It may be caused by excessive drinking of alcohol, or it may appear after an attack of hepatitis. It weakens the liver.

CONSTIPATION: Some people normally have three bowel movements a day, and others have only one bowel movement every ten days. Constipation occurs only when you have fewer bowel movements than what is normal for you or when the consistency of the stool changes and your stools are harder than usual. There is an astonishing variety in the frequency of bowel movements among different people and constipation, by itself, is not a sign of poor health.

CROHN'S DISEASE (REGIONAL ENTERITIS): This is an inflamed, ulcerating disease of the small intestine, or colon. It's an organic problem, but the symptoms can be made worse by gut reactions. Frequently, medication and even surgery are needed. Crohn's disease differs from ulcerative colitis because it is in a different part of the body's tissue. The small bowel is often involved in Crohn's disease, but never in ulcerative colitis.

DIGESTION: This term describes the whole process of food going from the intestinal tract and being broken down for absorption into the body for use as "fuel." Seven or eight major organs are involved in this process. It usually goes on all the time, but is less efficient when you're sick.

DIARRHEA: The most common cause of diarrhea is gut reactions. Any time the stool is more liquid than usual and you pass more than a pound of stool a day, you have what doctors interpret as diarrhea.

DIVERTICULOSIS: Sometimes, as a result of a chronically irritated colon or some other unusual strain, little fingerlike pouches form on the intestinal tract. This is known as diverticulosis. It may be one exception to the general rule that gut reactions don't cause organic disease.

DYSPHAGIA: This simply means "trouble in swallowing" and can be a functional disorder or come as a result of a tumor or other blockage in your throat, causing food to stick in your esophagus. You won't choke because the food isn't blocking your air passages, but some people get so much food stuck that it becomes impacted (packed in) and needs to be removed by a doctor.

ENEMA: This medical term means the forceful introduction of any material into the rectum, done to clear the colon of feces or other obstructions.

FART: This medical term describes the passing of air, or gas, through the rectum. The gas in your body is made up of air, plus several gaseous secretions such as methane.

HEARTBURN: When partly digested food "burps up" from the stomach back into the esophagus, the result is a burning sensation in the chest, known commonly as heartburn. Acid irritation, and possibly spasms, causes the burning feeling. It usually goes away by itself, and has nothing to do with your heart.

HEMORRHAGE: This term describes any abnormal and excessive bleeding from any part of the body, and it's a sure sign of organic disease. Never ignore blood in your stools or in your vomit, which could mean hemorrhage in the stomach or intestines. See your doctor at once.

HEPATITIS: This is a serious inflammation of the liver, usually caused by a virus.

HIATAL HERNIA: When the top of your stomach sticks up or "pouches" into your chest, you have a hiatal hernia. Part of the stomach is actually invading the chest, right under the breastbone. This may contribute to heartburn and perhaps some pain, and can be treated with medications.

HUNGER PAIN: It may be uncomfortable, but hunger pain is a sure sign of good health. It indicates increased activity of your intestines as they clamor for your attention and some food.

. . . ITIS: Any term ending in "itis" means inflammation. Irritation is always present, but you don't necessarily run a fever. Enteritis is an inflammation of the small bowel, hepatitis is liver inflammation, gastritis is an inflammation of the stomach, and so on.

JAUNDICE: This term indicates a yellowing of your skin and eyes, usually because of some liver disease. The jaundice is caused by a backup of bilirubin in your blood. Bilirubin is a chemical breakdown of bile which is normally excreted by the body through the liver; when the excretion slows down because of liver malfunction, the bilirubin overloads your bloodstream and gives your skin a yellowish tinge.

NAUSEA: This term describes the feeling of not wanting to digest your food, and preparing to expel it instead. It's the next step after anorexia (loss of appetite), and indicates a mental or physical insult to your body.

PAIN THRESHOLD: Every human has a different perception of pain, and the way you view pain is known as your pain threshold. People with high pain thresholds can take a lot of discomfort; people with low pain thresholds need more pain medication to feel comfortable. Your pain threshold is usually affected by your personality (a calm person can take more pain, for example), your environment (you withstand pain better if you're in a place you know and like), and the level of stress you're experiencing (things hurt more when you're upset).

PANCREATITIS: This is an inflammation of the pancreas, most commonly associated with alcohol abuse or gall bladder disease. It can cause severe abdominal pain and high fever, and frequently requires hospitalization.

REFLUX: When the muscles and nerves of your gastrointestinal tract are upset, they may work backwards and push food up and out of your mouth instead of down to your rectum. This is reflux. Most commonly it means that food in the stomach is "leaping up" back into the esophagus.

THROMBOSED: This term means "clotted with blood." When your hemorrhoids are blood clotted, you have "thrombosed hemorrhoids." It hurts, and is characterized by swelling of the affected area.

ULCER: Any breakdown of the lining of the intestinal tract is called an ulcer. Think of it as a sore anywhere in your guts. It can bleed and hurt, like a child's scraped knee.

ULCERATIVE COLITIS: This disease is the most common form of chronic colitis. It's an inflammation of the inner lining of the colon, and almost always involves the rectum. The disease is not a gut reaction; it's organic, and often causes bloody diarrhea. This disease is often confused with the closely related *ileitis*, which is inflammation of the lower half of the small intestine, or *ileum*. According to the National Foundation for Ileitis and Colitis, Inc., one out of every thousand adults in the United States now has ulcerative colitis, and the disease is rapidly increasing. The causes of the disease are unknown, but some researchers think it may be an allergic-like reaction in the tissues of the intestinal tract. Doctors often confuse the early symptoms of ulcerative colitis with gut reactions, and vice-versa, and often say stress plays a part in the disease. The Foundation declares that "Most physicians today doubt that emotional problems exclusively cause ileitis or colitis. On the other hand, most would agree that emotional factors influence the course of the disease—just as they influence the course of most other chronic diseases."

UMBILICUS: It's your navel. The term comes from umbilical cord, and is the point where the cord from the mother's placenta is joined to the fetus.

VOMIT: This describes the process of food "exploding" from your mouth, or being forcefully expelled. It indicates some sort of irritation in your esophagus or stomach, and isn't usually serious unless it is chronic.

Common Drugs Used by Gastroenterologists

This book has played down the use of drugs or medications for three reasons: (1) they are rarely useful in treating gut reactions; (2) it's dangerous and unwise to suggest that people can successfully self-medicate, or rely on drugs for help; and (3) the use of drugs can draw attention away from the patient's real responsibility, which is understanding and coping emotionally with gut reactions. Still, drugs are sometimes used in treating the irritable gut syndrome, and once in a while they can temporarily ease symptoms, so they deserve some mention here.

Any discussion of drugs must carry with it a two-pronged warning: know what they are, and know what they can do to your body. One little-known effect of drugs is the weird side reactions that may come when you mix them inside your body. Mixing tranquilizers with alcohol (also a drug) can kill, and mixing the common aspirin with any blood-thinning drug can set you up for hemorrhage.

The best way to protect yourself against drugs is to tell your doctor what drug you're taking so he won't prescribe one that "clashes." Don't take drugs prescribed for anyone else, and read the warnings printed on the labels of all prescription and over-the-counter drugs. To be sure, ask your pharmacist if you're in danger of "drug mixing" every time you buy a new drug. You should also be aware that some drugs interact poorly with certain foods. The food may impair the effectiveness of the drug, or speed up the way your body reacts to it. A good rule to remember is never take any drug with soda or acid fruit or vegetable juice; these drinks may make the drug dissolve too quickly and go into your stomach, rather than into your intestines, where they can be absorbed more easily. Follow your doctor's orders when he says, "Take the drug before (or after) a meal," and report any odd symptoms you feel after eating. "Food and Drug Interaction" by Phyllis Lehmann, available in a reprint from the FDA Consumer, March, 1978, is a good source to consult. You can get it from the U.S. Department of Health, Education and Welfare, Public Health Service, Food and Drug Administration, Office of Public Affairs, Washington, D. C. Ask for HEW Publication No. (FDA) 78-3070.

In the meantime, this brief list of common terms for drugs will give you some idea of what you might be putting into your body.

ANTACIDS: These are liquids or tablets used to neutralize acid in the gastrointestinal tract. Usually, they're made up of hydroxide mixed with aluminum, magnesium, or sodium bicarbonate.

ANTIBIOTICS: This family of drugs has been a boon to humanity, but they're dangerous when overused because resistant "bugs" or organisms can develop which may not be susceptible to any drug, or you can get an allergic reaction to the antibiotic itself. Antibiotics are used for infections of the gastrointestinal tract as well as for a host of other disorders.

ANTICHOLINERGICS: These are drugs that block the pathways of the involuntary nervous system. They affect the movements and secretions of the intestines and sometimes relieve pain and other gut symptoms.

ANTIDEPRESSANTS: These drugs, popularly known as "uppers," elevate moods and help alleviate depression.

ANTIDIARRHEAL AGENTS: As the name implies, these drugs slow down diarrhea.

CATHARTICS: This term indicates a laxative or a group of laxative-type drugs given to stimulate or enhance stool evacuation.

CIMETIDINE: This is a new, very potent antacid drug. It blocks the body's production of acids, and is useful in treating ulcer disease.

CORTISONE or STEROID DRUGS: These are "anti-inflammatory" drugs commonly used to treat colitis. They are related to cortisone, which is a natural secretion of the adrenal gland.

TRANQUILIZERS: These are the most commonly used and abused drugs—simply because they mask feelings of anxiety and fear, and temporarily make patients feel more in control of themselves. Tranquilizers work on your brain to make you feel calmer. They're also highly habit-forming.

Common Gastrointestinal Operations

Surgery should never be used to treat gut reactions. Now and then, however, you may find yourself with an organic disease—in addition to gut reactions—for which surgery is recommended. If so, you've got to make a complex and scary decision.

Whenever you've got reasonable doubts about the need for surgery, seek a second opinion in the form of advice from another doctor. Both doctors should know you're doing this.

Generally, find a surgeon through the recommendations made by your family doctor or gastroenterologist. Next, be careful in describing symptoms: are they clearly organic, like bleeding? Or is it heartburn, a symptom that could be either functional or organic? Also, is your organic disease treatable any other way? Gallstones or cancer almost always call for surgery. But if you have two ulcer attacks some surgeons will want to remove your stomach, while others may advise you to wait. That's when a second or even third opinion is useful.

Here's a list of the most common operative procedures performed on people who have organic gastrointestinal problems.

APPENDECTOMY: This is a routine operation for taking out an inflamed appendix. Recovery is usually rapid and you won't notice that the useless little bag is gone.

CHOLECYSTECTOMY: With this operation, your gallbladder is removed. You won't miss it; other organs take over the function of regulating bile.

COLECTOMY: This is an operation to remove part or all of the colon, or large intestine. The digestive process is temporarily slowed, but the body adjusts and can function quite well after recovery.

COLOSTOMY: In this operation the end part of the colon, or rectum, is removed. Afterwards, you must wear a bag to collect feces, because they come out of a hole in the abdominal wall, constructed by the surgeon as a replacement fecal exit.

GASTRECTOMY: Ulcer disease, bleeding, or cancer usually necessitates this operation, which is done to remove part or all of the stomach. Afterwards, most digestion takes place entirely in the small intestine.

HEMORRHOIDECTOMY: When the little veins in your anus are chronically and painfully swollen, your troublesome hemorrhoids are removed in this operation. Other veins then take over their job. This procedure gives the patient pain for several days, especially when moving the bowels. Expect a four- or five-day hospital stay and a recovery period of several weeks. Trouble can recur later, if other veins act up.

ILEOSTOMY: In this operation the small bowel, or ileum, is brought to the surface of the abdomen so digested material can go out of it, because the colon has been removed. Afterwards, patients must wear a bag to collect feces. The difference between an ileostomy and a colostomy is one of degree: in a colostomy, only part of the colon is removed; in an ileostomy, all of the colon is removed.

LAPAROTOMY: This medical term refers to any opening made on the abdomen for any surgical process. It indicates the beginning of a major operative procedure performed in the hospital with the patient under anesthesia.

POLYPECTOMY: A polyp is a growth that isn't supposed to be in your body, and doctors are fond of snipping them off because some polyps can be cancerous. This procedure usually involves the insertion of a tube into your rectum, which is maneuvered to the spot where the polyp is dangling like a grape hanging from a vine. The tube sometimes carries a tiny knife inside it, which pops out and snips off the polyp, which could be anywhere from a pea to a walnut in size. The polyp could also be burned off. This is a painful and risky surgical procedure usually done in the hospital, and performed so as to avoid more major surgery. Ask for heavy sedation and expect to be sore.

PYLOROPLASTY: This procedure to help the stomach empty more naturally—perhaps after it has been blocked by ulcers—is performed by opening up the end of the stomach.

VAGOTOMY: This operation involves cutting the nerves or nerve cords to the stomach to help heal ulcers. When the nerves are cut, acid secretion goes down and the healing process is aided. Usually a vagotomy and a pyloroplasty are performed at the same time.

It must be repeated that surgery is never a help in treating gut reactions. It's a last resort in the treatment of organic problems only. Sometimes doctors and patients confuse gut reactions with organic disease, and surgery might enter someone's mind as a possible cure. Don't buy it. If you have only gut reactions, you do have a disease, but surgery won't help. In the February, 1979, issue of *The Harvard Medical School Health Letter,* gut reactions were described this way:

"So here comes the question some of you have been waiting for: is the irritable bowel syndrome—or whatever you choose to call the problem—a *real disease?* If you insist that a disease must have anatomic changes that can be seen on X-ray or under the microscope, the answer may be 'no.' But if you are willing to accept—as most experts do—that motility problems can be just as real as deranged anatomy, then the answer must be 'yes.' ''

Yes, it's a disease. Yes, you can get rid of it.

Good luck.

Bibliography

Almy, Thomas P. and Bonkowsky, Herbert L. "Medicine in the 80's—Digestive Disease." *Drug Therapy* 33 (1980).

Almy, Thomas P. and Corson, John A. "Biofeedback—The Light at the End of the Tunnel?" *Gastroenterology* 76 (1979):874.

Barsky, Arthur J. III. "Patients Who Amplify Bodily Sensations." *Annals of Internal Medicine* 91 (1979):63.

Black, David. "Medicine and the Mind." *Playboy* magazine (April 1980):216.

Bond, John H. and Levitt, Michael D. "A Rational Approach to Intestinal Gas Problems." *Viewpoints on Digestive Disease* 9 (1977):2.

Burkitt, D. P. "Diet and Disease: Dietary Fibre." *Royal Society of Gastroenterology* 95 (1975):186.

Byrne, Jo-Anne. "Kids Learn to Control Some Ills with Self-hypnosis." *Atlanta Journal* (February 13, 1980):5B.

Carson, Ronald A. "What are Physicians For?" *Journal of the American Medical Association* 238 (1977):1029.

Cohen, Sidney and Snape, William J. "How Colonic Motility Differs in Normal Subjects and Patients with Irritable Bowel Syndrome." *Practical Gastroenterology* 3 (1979):21.

Chaudhary, Nazira and Truelove, S. C. "The Irritable Colon Syndrome." *The Quarterly Journal of Medicine* 31 (1962):307.

Dietschy, John M. "Advances in the Pharmacological Treatment of Gastrointestinal Disorders." *Drug Therapy* 33 (1978).

Donaldson, Robert M., Jr. "Diet and Gastrointestinal Disorders." *Gastroenterology* 52 (1967):897.

Drossman, Douglas A. "Irritable Bowel: Flexibility is the Key to Proper Management." *Modern Medicine* 48 (1980):26.

Drossman, Douglas A. "The Problem Patient." *Annals of Internal Medicine* 88 (1978):366.

Drossman, Douglas A. "Diagnosis of the Irritable Colon." *Annals of Internal Medicine* 90 (1979):431.

Drossbaum, Douglas A. and Powell, Don W. and Sessions, John T., Jr. "The Irritable Bowel Syndrome: A Challenge for the Physicians." *Current Concepts in Gastroenterology* 3 (1978):4.

Drossman, Douglas A. and Powell, Don W. and Sessions, John T., Jr. "The Irritable Bowel Syndrome." *Gastroenterology* 73 (1977):811.

Ferris, Timothy. "Hopeful Prophet Who Speaks for Human Aspiration." *Smithsonian* magazine (April 1980):127.

Fixx, James F. *The Complete Book of Running.* New York: Random House, 1977.

Glass, Jeffrey J. and Kirsner, Joseph B. "Drug-induced Gastrointestinal Disease—A Brief Overview." *Drug Therapy* (1976): 134.

Greenbaum, David S. "Intestinal Gas in Normal Subjects and Patients with Irritable Bowel Syndrome." *Practical Gastroenterology* 3 (1979):27.

Greenberg, Daniel S. "Washington Report—Nutrition: A Long Wait for a Little Advice." *New England Journal of Medicine* 302 (1980):535.

Groves, James E. "Taking Care of the Hateful Patient." *New England Journal of Medicine* 298 (1978):883.

Hogan, Walter J. "An Approach to the Medical Management of the Patient with Irritable Bowel Syndrome." *Practical Gastroenterology* 3 (1979):33.

Horrocks, James C. and DeDombal, F. T. "Clinical Presentation of Patients with 'Dyspersia.' " *Gut* 19 (1978):19.

Ingelfinger, Franz J. "How to Swallow and Belch and Cope with Heartburn." *Nutrition Today* 4 (1973).

Jukes, Thomas H. "The Organic Food Myth." *Journal of the American Medical Association* 230 (1974):276.

Kessel, Neil. "Reassurance." *The Lancet* 1 (1979):1128.

Kirsner, Joseph B. "The Irritable Bowel Syndrome— Some Personal Reflections." *Practical Gastroenterology* 3 (1979):50.

Knowles, John H. "Responsibility for Health." *Science* 198 (1977):1103.

Lehmann, Phyllis. "Food and Drug Interaction." FDA Consumer Reprint, U.S. Department of Health, Education and Welfare, Washington, D.C. (March 1978).

Mendeloff, Albert I. "Epidemiology of the Irritable Bowel Syndrome." *Practical Gastroenterology* 3 (1979):12.

Mendeloff, Albert I. "Dietary Fibre in Human Health." *New England Journal of Medicine* 297 (1977):811.

Mendeloff, Albert I. and Monk, Mary and Siegel, Charles I. and Lilienfeld, Abraham. "Illness Experience in Life Stresses in Patients with Irritable Colon and with Ulcerative Colitis." *New England Journal of Medicine* 282 (1970):14.

Menninger, W. Walter. "Caring as Part of Health Care Quality." *Journal of the American Medical Association* 234 (1975):836.

Morris, A. I. and Turnberg, L. A. "Surreptitious Laxative Abuse." *Gastroenterology* 77 (1979):80.

Palmer, Eddy D. *Functional Gastrointestinal Disease.* Baltimore: The Williams and Wilkins Press, 1967.

Panati, Charles. *Breakthroughs.* Boston: Houghton-Mifflin, 1980.

Pellegrino, Edmund D. *Humanism and the Physician.* Knoxville: The University of Tennessee Press, 1979.

Price, Steve F. and Smithson, Kenneth W. and Castell, Donald O. "Food Sensitivity in Reflux Esophagitis." *Gastroenterology* 75 (1978):240.

Rabkin, Judith G. and Struening, Elmer. "Life Events, Stress and Illness." *Science* 194 (1976):1013.

Rawson, M.D. "Cathartic Colon." *The Lancet* 1 (1966):1121.

Ritchie, James. "Pain and Irritable Bowel Syndrome." *Practical Gastroenterology* 3 (1979):17.

Salter, R. H. "What Should the Patient Eat?" *The Lancet* 1 (1969):879.

Scheibe, Donna. "Outlook on Life Determines How People Deal with Pain." *Atlanta Journal* (August 23, 1979):145.

Schuster, Marvin M. "Operant Conditioning in Gastrointestinal Dysfunction. *Hospital Practice* 9 (1974):135.

Schuster, Marvin M. "Irritable Bowel Syndrome—Introduction and Overview." *Practical Gastroenterology* 3 (1979):8.

Sheehan, George A. *Running and Being—The Total Experience.* New York: Simon and Schuster, 1978.

Silverberg, Mervin and Daum, Frederic. "Irritable Bowel Syndrome in Children and Adolescents." *Practical Gastroenterology* 3 (1979):25.

Soltoft, J. Karj B. and Gudmand, Hoyer E. and

Kristenson, E. and Welf, H. R. "A Double-Line Trial of the Effect of Wheat Bran on Symptoms of Irritable Bowel Syndrome." *The Lancet* 1 (1976):270.

Spiro, Howard M. "Pain and Perfectionism—The Physician and the 'Pain Patient.' " *New England Journal of Medicine* 4 (1976):829.

Sullivan, Mark A. and Cohen, Sidney and Snape, William J. "Colonic Myoelectrical Activity in Irritable-Bowel Syndrome." *New England Journal of Medicine* 298 (1978):878.

Swanson, David W. and Swenson, Wendell M. and Huizenga, Kenneth A. and Melson, Stephen J. "Persistent Nausea Without Organic Cause." *Mayo Clinic Proceedings*.

Thompson, W. Grant. *The Irritable Gut*. Baltimore: University Park Press, 1978.

Waller, Sheila L. and Misiewicz, J. J. "Prognosis in the Irritable Bowel Syndrome." *The Lancet* 2 (1969):753.

Whitehead, William E. and Schuster, Marvin M. "Psychological Management of the Irritable Bowel Syndrome." *Practical Gastroenterology* 3 (1979):33.

Wolf, Stewart G. *The Stomach*. New York: Oxford University Press, 1965.

Young, Stephen J. "Psychiatric Consideration in Irritable Bowel Syndrome." *Practical Gastroenterology* 3 (1979):29.

———. "Gas." *New England Journal of Medicine* 31 (1969):164.

———. "How Big Pains From Little Bellyaches Grow." *Medical World News* 521 (1973).

———. "The Colon and the Psyche." *The Lancet* 2 (1977):337.

———. "Dietary Fibre." *The Lancet* 2 (1977):337.

———. "Some Frequently Asked Questions About Ileitis and Colitis." *National Foundation for Ileitis and Colitis, Incorporated*. 295 Madison Avenue, New York, New York 10017.

————. "Unruly Guts." *The Lancet* 2 (1972):960.

————. "Management of the Irritable Bowel." *The Lancet* 2 (1978):557.

————. "Psychogenic Vomiting." *British Medical Journal* 2 (1968):344.

————. "Irritable Bowel Syndrome." *Harvard Medical School Health Letter* 4 (1979):4.

————. "Slower Recovery after Heart Attack Linked to Worrying." *Atlanta Journal* (January 30, 1980):6A.

————. "Belief in Happiness as Long Life Cause is Bolstered by Study." *Wall Street Journal* (May 6, 1979):18.

————. "Psychosomatic Medicine Finds Why Work Can Be Sickening." *New York Times* (February 3, 1980):22E.